A Volume in The Laboratory Animal Pocket Reference Series

The Laboratory
CANINE

The Laboratory Animal Pocket Reference Series

Series Editor
Mark A. Suckow, D.V.M.
Freimann Life Science Center
University of Notre Dame
Notre Dame, IN

Published Titles

The Laboratory Canine
The Laboratory Cat
The Laboratory Guinea Pig
The Laboratory Hamster and Gerbil
The Laboratory Mouse
The Laboratory Nonhuman Primate
The Laboratory Rabbit
The Laboratory Rat
The Laboratory Small Ruminant
The Laboratory Swine

A Volume in The Laboratory Animal Pocket Reference Series

The Laboratory
CANINE

Garrett Field
Diplomate ACLAM
Eli Lilly and Company
Indianapolis, Indiana

Todd A. Jackson
Diplomate ACLAM
Bristol-Myers Squibb
Evansville, Indiana

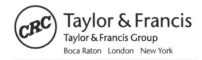

Taylor & Francis
Taylor & Francis Group
Boca Raton   London   New York

CRC is an imprint of the Taylor & Francis Group,
an informa business

CRC Press
Taylor & Francis Group
6000 Broken Sound Parkway NW, Suite 300
Boca Raton, FL 33487-2742

© 2007 by Taylor & Francis Group, LLC
CRC Press is an imprint of Taylor & Francis Group, an Informa business

No claim to original U.S. Government works
Printed in the United States of America on acid-free paper
10 9 8 7 6 5 4 3 2 1

International Standard Book Number-10: 0-8493-2893-4 (Softcover)
International Standard Book Number-13: 978-0-8493-2893-0 (Softcover)

Library of Congress Cataloging-in-Publication Data

Field, Garrett.
  The laboratory canine / Garrett Field and Todd A. Jackson.
    p. cm. – (Laboratory animal pocket reference series)
  ISBN 0-8493-2893-4 (alk. paper)
  1. Dogs as laboratory animals. I. Jackson, Todd A. II. Title. III. Series.

  SF407.D6F54 2006
  636.7'0885--dc22   2006045553

Visit the Taylor & Francis Web site at
http://www.taylorandfrancis.com

and the CRC Press Web site at
http://www.crcpress.com

dedication

This book is dedicated to the Animal Caretakers who provide daily care for canines used in research. It is through their caring, dedication, and patience that we have the ability and privilege to work with these wonderful animals. I also wish to thank my wife Deborah, for her spirit, love, support, and editorial assistance with this book. My parents, Virginia and William, my siblings, and my professional colleagues helped me become a better person and professional. Lastly, my pet dogs serve as a constant reminder of the gentle nature of the species and inspire me to do my best in caring for their canine relatives every day.

Garrett Field, D.V.M.

Thanks to my family, Lois, Ellen, and Sam, for their support. Thanks also to the long list of mentors who have helped guide my training, starting with Weyman B. Salmon, D.V.M., better known to his friends and clients simply as "Doc."

Todd Jackson, D.V.M.

the authors

Garrett Field, D.V.M., is Principal Research Veterinarian at Eli Lilly and Company, Indianapolis, Indiana. Dr. Field earned his Doctor of Veterinary Medicine from Louisiana State University in 1988 and completed a postdoctoral residency in laboratory animal medicine at the University of Michigan in 1991. He is a Diplomate of the American College of Laboratory Animal Medicine. Dr. Field has more than 20 years experience in biomedical research in the public and private sectors.

Todd Jackson, D.V.M., is Director of Veterinary Sciences at Bristol-Myers Squibb, Evansville, Indiana. Dr. Jackson earned his Doctor of Veterinary Medicine from Purdue University in 1990 and completed a postdoctoral residency in laboratory animal medicine at the University of Michigan in 1996. He is a Diplomate of the American College of Laboratory Animal Medicine. Dr. Jackson has more than 10 years experience in biomedical research in the public and private sectors.

The authors' proceeds will be donated and split equally between the ACLAM Foundation and the AALAS Foundation for use in funding research, education, and training of Animal Care Technicians in laboratory animal science.

acknowledgments

The authors graciously acknowledge Dr. Gerald Smith for his thoughtful review and editorial suggestions and Dr. Jodi Carlson for her beautiful illustrations. They helped make the book much better.

preface

The use of laboratory animals, including canines, continues to be an important part of biomedical research. Individuals caring for and working with dogs in a research setting are charged with broad responsibilities including animal husbandry, social enrichment, animal facility management, veterinary care, regulatory compliance, and performing the various technical procedures required as part of the individual research projects performed. This handbook was prepared to serve as a quick reference source for those individuals charged with the care and use of canines in a research setting. It should be particularly valuable for those individuals with less training or experience with laboratory canines and institutions just beginning programs to use and care for laboratory dogs.

This handbook is organized into six chapters: "Important Biological Features" (Chapter 1), "Husbandry" (Chapter 2), "Management" (Chapter 3), "Veterinary Care" (Chapter 4), "Experimental Methodology" (Chapter 5), and "Resources" (Chapter 6). Basic information, standard practices, and common procedures are detailed within the book. Literature references, best practices of other institutions, and the authors' knowledge and experience were source material for the book. It is not the intention of the authors to provide an exhaustive review of the subject material, but rather to provide a handbook that is useful as a quick reference. The reader should consult other more detailed reviews for individual topics or content beyond the scope of this book.

Dogs have a long history of use in research and, like so many other animals, have contributed enormously to the health and welfare of both humans and animals. Dogs are also a highly visible species in the eyes of the public and regulators. For these reasons and others, it is important that individuals working with laboratory canines have the proper training and experience. Working under the direction of a veterinarian experienced in laboratory animal medicine and canine medicine is highly recommended.

contents

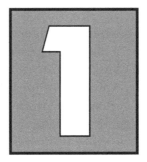

important biological features

Dogs have a long history of use in research and, like so many other animals, have contributed enormously to the health and welfare of both humans and animals. Dating back to the 1600s, research conducted by William Harvey on cardiac movement and later research by Louis Pasteur and Anton Pavlov included the use of dogs. Early factors accounting for their use included their gentle nature as a companion animal, size, availability, ease of care, and anatomical and physiological similarities to man. Contemporary use of dogs has evolved based on the discovery of dogs demonstrating congenital, spontaneous, or inducible models of human diseases. Beagles are the primary breed of dog used for research, and random-source dogs used in research are most commonly mongrels or larger breeds such as German shepherds and Labrador retrievers.[1,2] The use of dogs in research has steadily declined from a peak of 211,104 in 1979 to 64,932 in 2004 (U.S. Department of Agriculture).[3]

origin of the dog

The domestic dog, *Canis familiaris*, is a member of the order Carnivora and the family Canidae, which includes a distinct group of dog- and fox-like animals distributed worldwide. Closely related to domestic dogs are the gray and red wolves (*Canis lupus* and *Canis rufus*), coyotes (*Canis laterans*), and four species of jackals (*Canis aureus*, *Canis adustus*, *Canis mesomelas*, and *Canis simensis*). Other distant family members include dingoes (*Canis lupus dingo*) and multiple species of fox (*Vulpes* sp.). Interbreeding is possible between close family members of the domestic dog (dog and wolf, dog and coyote). Based on fossil evidence, the first dogs were introduced into North America prior to 8400 B.C. when they migrated across the Bering Strait.

Domestication of dogs, purportedly the first species of animal domesticated by man, is believed to have occurred in Asia around 10,000 B.C. when wolves were initially domesticated. Domestication is thought to have occurred in an unplanned manner as scraps of food were scavenged from village waste dumps then shared by man with dogs. Later, a mutually beneficial working relationship developed as man was eventually recognized as the better hunter-provider through the use of weapons and traps. Subsequently, one surmises, dogs were adopted and tamed and then became active participants in the hunt, tracking, flushing, isolating, and even capturing game for their masters.

The further domestication of dogs was a troubled journey. While some ancient cultures elevated dogs to cult (Egypt, Persia) or mythological status (Greece), where killing a dog was a corporal crime and dogs were entombed with their masters, other cultures consumed dogs as a food source (still practiced). In Rome, hunting dogs were highly esteemed, ferocious guard dogs were common, and others were used in war as messengers and for attack. During the medieval period, dogs fell into disfavor and were abandoned to fend for themselves, hunting in packs. During the Middle Ages and Renaissance periods, with prosperity and cultural shifts, dogs again became important as working dogs and specialization began in earnest. Hunting, herding, guarding, and use in warfare increased. Later, dogs filtered into the middle class, as companions and as subjects of art.[4-6]

In 1859, the earliest dog show is reported to have occurred, reflecting renewed breed specialization and the growing appreciation for dogs as intelligent, attractive animals. In 1873, the English Kennel Club was founded, followed by the founding of the American Kennel Club in 1884. Concurrently, concerns over animal welfare and cruelty to animals increased and common practices were abolished, such as ear docking in England. Early laws to protect animals from careless owners as well as to protect those used in research were passed. With the advent of the 20th century and beyond, dogs were well integrated into society as traditional working dogs, as companion dogs, and in new areas of specialization. For example, dogs now work in search and rescue, in law enforcement, as service dogs for the handicapped, as actors, and in research as models of disease. It is in this latter role that dogs serve the noblest of roles for mankind, even preceding man into space.

dog breeds

Worldwide there are about 320 breeds of dogs. A general classification of dogs includes sporting dogs, hounds, working dogs, terriers, toy dogs, and nonsporting dogs. Contributing to the development of local breeds of particular use was the geographic isolation of ancestral world cultures. While the Chinese were probably the earliest breeders of purebred dogs, the concept of breed was initially defined by the Arab culture.

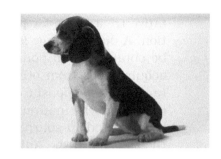

Figure 1.1 An adult pedigreed beagle. (Courtesy of Roberta Scipioni Ball, Marshall Farms)

The primary dog breeds used in research are beagles (Figure 1.1) and a variety of pedigreed hound-type dogs (Figures 1.2 and 1.3) collectively referred to as mongrels. When used for breeding purposes, a male dog is referred to as a **sire** or **stud,** a female dog is referred to as a **dam** or **bitch,** and an immature dog is called a **puppy.**

Dogs used in research are generally classified as either purpose-bred or random-source. Similar to other lab animal species (rodents, rabbits, etc.), purpose-bred dogs are bred specifically for biomedical research. The advantages include improved health status, better

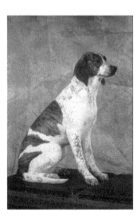

Figure 1.2 An adult pedigreed mongrel. (Courtesy of Roberta Scipioni Ball, Marshall Farms)

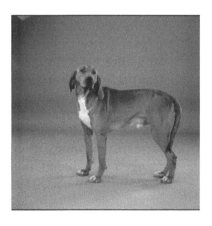

Figure 1.3 An adult pedigreed mongrel. (Courtesy of Roberta Scipioni Ball, Marshall Farms)

veterinary care including a known vaccination history and preventative treatments for parasites, a pedigree, and improved socialization. A disadvantage is their higher cost. Random-source dogs may be obtained from pounds and shelters or from dealers who legally acquire dogs from other sources. Their advantages and disadvantages are the opposite of purpose-bred dogs. Although it is rare, concern about the inadvertent use of pet dogs in research will remain as long as random-source dogs are still used. This issue was seminal in the passage of the Animal Welfare Act, and more states are legislating against the use of random-source dogs.[1,2,4,5]

dog behavior

Dog behavior is commonly divided into genetically defined (instinctual) and learned behavior. To better understand their behavior, one needs to understand their early origins as well as their subsequent domestication by man. One should remain cognizant of their origins when working with dogs or when attempting to assess or modify their behavior (tame/train) and not be overly anthropomorphic and apply human standards. Despite some owners' personal beliefs to the contrary, dogs lack the higher cognitive functions and language of man.

As **carnivores,** by definition, dogs are of an order of mammals that are flesh-eating creatures. Their various physiognomies include robust canine teeth for cutting and tearing, molar teeth for crushing and cutting, limbs adapted for endurance, toes with claws, and a keen sense of smell and visual acuity for predation/hunting. As predators, they hunt in packs, demonstrating intelligence and order. The pack mentality is part of their social order, characterized by a strong sense of family, a social and friendly nature, and a dedication to caring for their young.

Domestication by man was a practical extension of the canine social order, where the pack mentality, social organization, and hierarchy now included man. In this new arrangement, the shared interests and similarities between the species (i.e., hunting, intelligence, social order, affectionate nature, etc.) were important, as was the clear choice by dogs of the establishment of man's dominance in the new order.

While there are many breed and individual variations, modern dogs' ability to be domesticated is primarily based on some fundamental behavioral characteristics. In particular, these include dogs' intelligence; their docile, playful, tolerant, and participatory nature;

their ability to be trained; and their strong social nature. However, dogs are capable of exhibiting a wide range of other, less desirable behaviors that should be clearly understood and recognized when working in a research environment. Fear, anxiety, aggression, passivity, submissiveness, protectiveness, defensiveness, and complex abnormal psychologies are behaviors one expects to encounter in research based on individual dogs' variation or due to inadequate socialization, experimental manipulation, the development of disease, or inadequate care.

Communication between dogs occurs through a variety of complex olfactory, visual, auditory, vocalization, and tactile signals. The **olfactory sense** is the most developed sense in dogs, and scent marking and detection occurs in a number of ways. Dogs commonly urinate to mark their territory. Rubbing against or scratching surfaces is another means of imparting scent odors. Some experts believe that dogs vigorously scratching the ground following elimination or wagging their tails are means of spreading their scent. Similarly dogs' circling their sleep area prior to bedding down is a means of defining their sleep area by ritualistically tromping down the "vegetation" to define and mark their beds. Glands near the anus contain foul smelling secretions used for marking and are expressed when dogs are stressed or fearful. Through a combination of a wet nose to trap and absorb odors and a marvelously developed olfactory organ, the ability of dogs to detect odors is highly developed. Sniffing is a key part of a dog's greeting to assess other dogs, humans, and their environment.

Visual cues related to posture, position of body parts, and overall presentation by which dogs communicate are well described.[6–8] Classically, a wagging tail suggests joy; a tail down or between the legs suggests insecurity or fear; ears up suggests alertness; ears forward suggests alarm; lips raised and drawn back suggests fear and aggression. Trained and experienced lab personnel understand and distinguish these cues which are critical to ensure safe handling during experimental manipulation, to recognize often subtle, study/compound-related affects, or to recognize adverse clinical signs due to spontaneous illness unrelated to research use. While vision is predominantly limited to black and white, dogs have a greater ability to see in the dark than man.

Dogs have a highly developed sense of **hearing.** They are capable of hearing high-frequency sounds far above those of humans, up to and including the ultrasonic range. Dogs are able to discriminate well between different sounds and the direction from which sounds emanate. **Vocalizations** (barking, growling, and howling) communicate a wide range of emotions.[9]

Socialization occurs early in a dog's life, with most experts agreeing that the first 16 weeks are critical to establishing the dog's future behavior. Early socialization with conspecifics during rearing should be followed by earnest socialization activities with humans by 5 to 9 weeks of age. Therefore it is of paramount importance that dogs be adequately socialized by the breeder. The consequences of doing otherwise are dire. Contrary to domestic cats, which have historically tended to live isolated existences, fail to recognize another as their leader, and are arguably less trainable than dogs, dogs are eminently trainable.[4,6–9]

Enrichment may be viewed not only as an important part of the early socialization process for dogs, but also as an ongoing program critical to sustained socialization and overall health and wellness. While it's somewhat impractical to offer the degree and types of interactions and stimulation to dogs used in research as one would with pet dogs, the principles remain the same and serve as the basis for a rewarding enrichment program for dogs that produces happy, stable, and healthy dogs for research. An abundance of publications exist on dog behavior and readers are encouraged to consult other sources for additional information.

anatomic and physiologic features of dogs

Detailed dog anatomy texts are available, such as *Miller's Anatomy of the Dog* (W.B. Saunders, Philadelphia).[4] The phylogenetic classification of dogs is:

Kingdom	Chordata
Phylum	Vertebrata
Class	Mammalia
Order	Carnivora
Family	Canidae
Genus	Canis
Species	Familiaris

Thus the genus and species designation of the dog is *Canis familiaris*.

The adult dental formula of dogs is $2 \times ($incisors$_{3/3}$, canines$_{1/1}$, premolars$_{4/4}$, molars$_{2/3}) = 42$. Eruption of the second, permanent set of (adult) teeth occurs between 2 and 7 months of age. Eruption of the first set of puppy (deciduous) teeth occurs by 2 months of age and does not include molars. The puppy dental formula of dogs is 2 × (incisors$_{3/3}$, canines$_{1/1}$, premolars$_{3/3}$) = 28. Dogs have specialized shearing-cutting teeth, the upper fourth premolars, called the carnassial teeth.

The average adult canine skeleton contains 320 bones, including the sesamoid bones. Not included are the dewclaws, which are variably developed in many breeds, and the os penis (baculum), the boney structure in the male dog's penis. The vertebral formula in dogs is cervical (7), thoracic (13), lumbar (7), sacral (3), caudal (20) = 50.[10]

Dogs have five digits on the forepaws and four digits on the hind paws. The first digit on each paw (numbered from medial to lateral) is generally rudimentary. On the hind paw, the first medial digit is called the dewclaw.[10]

Dog lungs are divided into left and right halves. The left lung is divided into two lobes: the left cranial and caudal lobes. The left cranial lobe is further divided into cranial and caudal parts separated by an incomplete fissure. The right lung is divided into four lobes: the right cranial, middle, accessory, and caudal lobes.[11]

Dog livers are divided into four lobes: the left hepatic, right hepatic, quadrate, and caudate lobes. The left and right hepatic lobes are divided into medial and lateral lobes. The caudate lobe is divided into the caudate and papillary processes. The left hepatic lobe comprises from one-third to one-half of the total liver mass. The gall bladder lies between the quadrate and right medial hepatic lobes.[12]

Dog taste buds are located within the gustatory (fungiform, vallate, and foliate) sensory papillae distributed across the tongue. Sensitivity to sweet taste is limited to the rostral margins and tip of the tongue, while sour taste sensitivity is distributed over the dorsal tongue. Salt sensitivity is primarily along the tongue margins and a narrow transverse area across the back of the tongue, although some reports describe dogs as insensitive to salt. Dogs have a relatively short alimentary tract and a small cecum.[9,12]

Dogs have a well-developed third eyelid, the nictitating membrane. It arises from the ventromedial aspect of the eye and is generally inapparent. It provides physical protection to the eye and contains glands that contribute to normal tear production.[13]

Dog vision is predominately black and white with minimal color vision (violet and yellow-green), attributable to the great preponderance of photoreceptors being rods (95%) versus cones (5%). Dogs can see well at lower levels of illumination compared to humans because light is reflected by a dog's tapetum lucidum, an area in the choriod (vascular) layer of the eye. Puppy eyes open around 12 to 15 days of age.[9,13]

The diploid number of chromosomes in dogs is 78. There are 38 homologous pairs of autosomes and 2 sex chromosomes.

Gestation in dogs is about 60 to 65 days. Controlled breeding programs have resulted in year-round breeding of dogs versus the seasonal monestrous breeding patterns previously observed.[18] Litter size is variable by breed.

normative values of the dog

Normative values listed represent typical values for the species and should be used as guidelines. Basic biological parameters (Table 1.1), hematology (Table 1.2), chemistry (Table 1.3), coagulation (Table 1.4), cerebrospinal fluid (Table 1.5), cardiovascular and respiratory (Table 1.6), urine (Table 1.7), synovial fluid (Table 1.8), and reproductive (Table 1.9) data and a growth chart (Table 1.10) are provided. Tables 1.2, 1.3, and 1.10 are data primarily from a commercial beagle colony. The other tables' data are not breed specific. It is highly desirable to establish in-house normative values, which can be customized to account for age, sex, breed, and laboratory variations.

TABLE 1.1: BASIC BIOLOGICAL PARAMETERS OF THE DOG

Parameter	Typical values	References
Diploid chromosome number	78	1
Life span (years)	12	1
Body weight (lb.) Beagle Mongrel	15–35 45–90	
Body temperature (°F)	101.5 ± 1.5	1
Metabolic energy requirement (kcal/kg/day) Adult	65	19
Food intake (g/day)	300–500	1
Water intake (ml/kg/day)	25–35	1
Fecal output (g feces/kg body weight/day)	8.5 ± 1.1	15
Dental formula Juvenile	$2 \times \left(\begin{array}{l} \text{Incisors}_{3/3}, \text{ canine}_{1/1}, \text{premolars}_{3/3} \\ = 28 \end{array} \right)$	12
Adult	$2 \times \left(\begin{array}{l} \text{Incisors}_{3/3}, \text{ canine}_{1/1}, \text{ premolars}_{4/4}, \\ \text{molars}_{2/3} = 42 \end{array} \right)$	

TABLE **1.2:** HEMATOLOGIC VALUES OF THE DOG

Parameter	Typical values		Range	References
	Male	**Female**	**Range**	**References**
Hematocrit (%)	49.4 ± 3.5	48.6 ± 4.0	34–58	
Red blood cells (10^6/μl)	7.1 ± 0.5	7.0 ± 0.6	5.0–8.5	
White blood cells (10^3/μl)	13.5 ± 3.7	14.3 ± 4.1	6.0–19.5	
Hemoglobin (g/dl)	16.9 ± 1.3	16.5 ± 1.6	11.9–18.9	
Neutrophils (10^3/μl)	8.6 ± 3.0	9.1 ± 3.3	1.8–16.6	
Lymphocytes (10^3/μl)	3.5 ± 0.8	3.7 ± 0.8	0.7–11.7	
Eosinophils (10^3/μl)	0.4 ± 0.2	0.4 ± 0.2	0–1.9	
Basophils (10^3/μl)	0.1 ± 0.1	0.1 ± 0.1	0–0.6	
Monocytes (10^3/μl)	0.8 ± 0.3	0.8 ± 0.4	0–2.7	
Platelets (10^3/μl)	342.8 ± 76.2	435.0 ± 122.2	140–850	
Reticulocytes (%)	0–1.5%	0–1.5%	0–1.5	
Mean corpuscular volume (MCV) (fl)	69.8 ± 2.1	69.5 ± 2.2	60–80	
Mean corpuscular hemoglobin concentration (MCHC) (g/dl)	34.1± 0.7	33.9 ± 1.1	25–38	
Mean corpuscular hemoglobin (MCH) (pg)	23.8 ± 0.9	23.6 ± 1.1	17.5–28	
Blood volume (ml/kg)			76.5–107.3	1
Plasma volume (ml/kg)			43.7–73.0	1
Erythrocyte life span (days)	110	110	100–120	14

Data primarily from commercial beagle colony (courtesy of Roberta Scipioni Ball, Marshall Farms) and as otherwise referenced.

TABLE 1.3: CLINICAL CHEMISTRY VALUES OF THE DOG

Parameter	Typical values Male	Typical values Female	Range	References
Total protein (mg/dl)	6.2 ± 0.4	6.1 ± 0.4	5.6–7.1	
Globulin (mg/dl)	2.6 ± 0.3	2.5 ± 0.3	1.9–3.6	
Albumin (mg/dl)	4.3 ± 4.8	4.0 ± 3.6	3.1–4.1	
Amylase (U/l)	743.4 ± 135.4	532.4 ± 109.7	286–1124	
Alkaline phosphatase (U/l)	63.2 ± 31.0	62.0 ± 36.1	12–122	
L-lactate dehydrogenase (LDH) (U/l)	53.0 ± 23.9	58.0 ± 38.0	45–233	2, 16
Aspartate transaminase (AST)/serum glutamic-oxaloacetic transaminase (SGOT) (U/l)	38.1 ± 10.2	35.2 ± 8.4	16–50	
Creatine kinase (U/l)	240.3 ± 238.7	190.9 ± 104.9	58–241	
Alanine transaminase (ALT)/serum glutamic-pyruvic transaminase (SGPT) (U/l)	48.3 ± 14.1	43.3 ± 16.7	25–106	
γ-glutamyltransferase (GGT) (U/l)	3.0 ± 0.1	3.1 ± 0.6	0–10	
Blood urea nitrogen (mg/dl)	22.1 ± 5.5	21.9 ± 6.9	8–30	
Creatinine (mg/dl)	0.8 ± 0.2	0.8 ± 0.3	0.5–1.3	
Glucose (mg/dl)	87.4 ± 13.3	85.2 ± 15.2	60–120	
Calcium (mg/dl)	10.6 ± 0.4	10.8 ± 0.4	7.2–12.8	
Magnesium (mEq/l)	1.7 ± 0.1	1.7 ± 0.1	1.4–1.8	
Phosphorous (mg/dl)	5.3 ± 0.9	5.3 ± 0.9	3.3–6.0	
Total bilirubin (mg/dl)	0.1 ± 0.0	0.1 ± 0.0	0.1–0.2	
Uric acid (mg/dl)	1.15 ± 1.43	1.06 ± 1.45	0–2.0	2, 16
Triglycerides (mg/dl)	58.0 ± 19.0	65.0 ± 22.9		2
Cholesterol (mg/dl)	184.1 ± 32.7	211.8 ± 48.8	124–335	
Sodium (mEq/l)	148.3 ± 1.9	149.1 ± 1.8	142–151	
Potassium (mEq/l)	4.9 ± 0.3	5.0 ± 0.4	3.9–5.3	
Chloride (mEq/l)	110.6 ± 1.9	111.1 ± 2.9	107–117	
Bicarbonate (mEq/l)	21.9 ± 2.7	22.5 ± 2.4	15–25	
Anion gap (mEq/l)	20.7 ± 2.4	20.5 ± 2.4	13–25	

Data primarily from commercial beagle colony (courtesy of Roberta Scipioni Ball, Marshall Farms) and as otherwise referenced.

TABLE 1.4: COAGULATION VALUES OF THE DOG

Parameter	Typical values	References
Bleeding time (minutes)	1–5	14
Clotting time		14
Whole blood (minutes)	3–13	
Activated clotting time (ACT, seconds)	60–100	
Clotting time (plasma, seconds)		14
Partial thromboplastic time (APTT)	11–19	
Prothrombin time (OSPT/PT)	5–12	
Thrombin time (TCT)	3–8	
Fibrin degradation products (FDP, μg/ml)	<32	14

TABLE 1.5: CEREBROSPINAL FLUID VALUES OF THE DOG

Parameter	Typical values	References
Red blood cells (cells/μl)	0–5	16
White blood cells (cells/μl)	0–5	16
Protein (mg/dl)	<25	16
Specific gravity	1.003–1.006	16
Glucose (mg/dl)	40–80	16
Color	Colorless	16
Turbidity	Clear	16

TABLE 1.6: VALUES FOR CARDIOVASCULAR AND RESPIRATORY FUNCTION OF THE DOG

Parameter	Typical values	References
Respiratory rate (breaths/minute)	20–40	2
Heart rate (beats/minute)	70–180	2
Blood gas values		2, 15
Arterial pO_2 (mm Hg)	92.1±1 5.6	
Arterial pCO_2 (mm Hg)	36.8 ± 3.0	
Arterial HCO_3 (mmol/l)	22.1 ± 1.7	
Arterial base excess (mEq/l)	–3 to +3	
Blood gas values		2, 15
Venous pO_2 (mm Hg)	52.1 ± 2.11	
Venous pCO_2 (mm Hg)	36.6 ± 1.21	
Venous HCO_3 (mmol/l)	22.3 ± 0.43	
Arterial blood pressure (mm Hg)		1
Systolic	95–136	
Diastolic	43–66	
Arterial blood pH	7.30–7.43	2
Capillary refill time (seconds)	< 1.5	2

TABLE 1.7: URINE VALUES OF THE DOG

Parameter	Typical values	References
Specific gravity	1.015–1.045	16
pH	6.0–7.0	16, 17
Volume (ml/kg/day)	24–40	17
Color	Yellow–amber	17
Appearance	Clear	17
Protein	0–trace	16
Glucose	Negative	16, 17
Ketones	Negative	16, 17
Urobilinogen	Negative	16
Bilirubin	0–trace	16, 17
Cells (cells/hpf)	0–8 red blood cells or white blood cells	17
Crystals/casts (cells/lpf)	0–2 hyaline or granular casts	17

hpf, high-power field; lpf, low-power field.

TABLE 1.8: SYNOVIAL FLUID VALUES OF THE DOG

Parameter	Typical values	References
Amount (ml)	0.01–1.0	16
pH	7.0–7.8	16
Erythrocytes ($\times 10^3$ µl)	0–320	16
Total white blood cells ($\times 10^3$ µl)	0–2.9	16
Neutrophils/µl	0–32	16
Monocytes/µl	0–838	16
Lymphocytes/µl	0–2436	16
Color	Yellow–amber	16
Mucin clot	Tight, ropy clump Clear supernatant	16

TABLE **1.9:** REPRODUCTIVE VALUES OF THE DOG

Parameter	Typical values	References
Gestation period (days)	59–68	1
Litter size (varies by breed)	1–12	1
Pseudopregnancy (days)	Common, 60	1
Estrus duration (days)	9–10	1
Breeding season (frequency/year)	Year-round	1, 18
Sexual maturity (months)		1
Male	6–12	
Female	6–12	
Breeding life (years)		1
Male	6	
Female	6	
Weaning age (weeks)	6–8	
Semen volume (ml/10–34 lb. dog)	2.4 ± 0.3	15
Sperm concentration (× 10^6/ml)	209 ± 42	15
Total sperm (× 10^6/ml)	400 ± 110	15

TABLE **1.10:** BEAGLE GROWTH CURVE

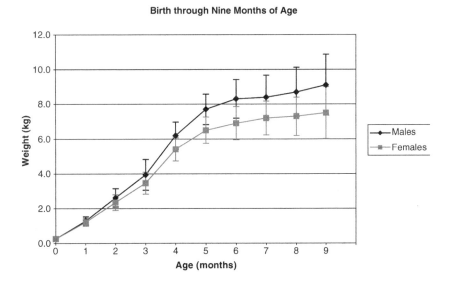

Data from commercial beagle colony (courtesy of Roberta Scipioni Ball, Marshall Farms).

references

1. Ringler, D.H. and Peter, G.K., Dogs and cats as laboratory animals, in *Laboratory Animal Medicine*, Fox, J.G., Cohen, B.J., and Loew, F.M., eds., Academic Press, San Diego, 1984, chap. 9.

2. Dysko, R.C., Nemzek, J.A., Levin, S.I., DeMarco, G.J., and Moalli, M.R., Biology and diseases of dogs, in *Laboratory Animal Medicine*, 2nd ed., Fox, J.G., Anderson, L.C., Loew, F.M., and Quimby, F.W., eds., Academic Press, San Diego, 2002, chap. 11.

3. *FY 2004 AWA Inspections*, Animal Care, Animal and Plant Health Inspection Service, U.S. Department of Agriculture, Washington, DC.

4. Evans, H.E., Classification and natural history of the dog, in *Miller's Anatomy of the Dog*, Evans, H.E. and Christensen, G.C., eds., W.B. Saunders, Philadelphia, 1979, chap. 1.

5. Pugnetti, G., Introduction, in *Simon and Schuster's Guide to Dogs*, Schuler, E.M., ed., Simon and Shuster, New York, 1980.

6. Coppinger, R. and Coppinger, L.C., *Dogs: A Startling New Understanding of Canine Origin, Behavior and Evolution*, Simon and Schuster, New York, 2001.

7. Monks of New Skete, Opening up to the world, in *The Art of Raising a Puppy*, Little, Brown, Boston, 1991, chap. 5.

8. Committee on Dogs of the Institute for Laboratory Animal Resources, *Laboratory Animal Management: Dogs*, National Academy Press, Washington, DC, 1994.

9. Joint Working Group on Refinement, Refining dog husbandry and care, *Lab. Anim.*, 38 (suppl. 1), 1, 2004.

10. Evans, H.E. and Christensen, G.C., The skeleton, in *Miller's Anatomy of the Dog*, Evans, H.E. and Christensen, G.C., eds., W.B. Saunders, Philadelphia, 1979, chap. 4.

11. Evans, H.E. and Christensen, G.C., The respiratory apparatus, in *Miller's Anatomy of the Dog*, Evans, H.E. and Christensen, G.C., eds., W.B. Saunders, Philadelphia, 1979, chap. 8.

12. Evans, H.E. and Christensen, G.C., The digestive apparatus and abdomen, in *Miller's Anatomy of the Dog*, Evans, H.E. and Christensen, G.C., eds., W.B. Saunders, Philadelphia, 1979, chap. 7.

13. Pollock, R.V.H., The eye, in *Miller's Anatomy of the Dog*, Evans, H.E. and Christensen, G.C., eds., W.B. Saunders, Philadelphia, 1979, chap. 20.

14. Duncan, J.R. and Prosse, K.W., *Veterinary Laboratory Medicine Clinical Pathology*, 2nd ed., Iowa State University Press, Ames, 1986.

15. Bonagura, J.D., *Kirk's Veterinary Therapy XIII: Small Animal Practice*, W.B. Saunders, Philadelphia, 2000.

16. Slatter, D., *Textbook of Small Animal Surgery*, 2nd ed., W.B. Saunders, Philadelphia, 1993.

17. Kirk, R.W. and Bistner, S.I., *Handbook of Veterinary Procedures & Emergency Treatment*, 4th ed., W.B. Saunders, Philadelphia, 1985.

18. McDonald, L.E., *Veterinary Endocrinology and Reproduction*, Lea & Febiger, Philadelphia, 377, 1969.

19. Kahn, C.M. and Line, S., eds., *The Merck Veterinary Manual*, 9th ed., Merck & Co., Whitehouse Station, 2005.

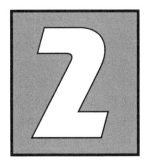

husbandry

Canines are generally easy to handle and house compared with other species, and many entry-level animal caretakers have prior experience handling pet dogs. However, good husbandry programs for dogs with adequate facilities and thorough staff training programs remain critically important. Dogs are a high profile species with regulatory agencies and in the eyes of the public. Lapses in canine husbandry programs can have serious consequences.

housing

Facility Design Considerations

Whenever possible, animal facilities should be designed to house dogs in an area separate from other, quieter species. Noise from barking dogs can be stressful to rabbits and rodents. Dog rooms should also be distanced from office areas for the comfort of people working in the facility.

Dog housing areas should be located near to the procedure areas where they will be used. The transportation of dogs through public corridors should be avoided.

Facilities housing dogs should have appropriate support space for their veterinary medical care. This includes a stocked and equipped pharmacy, treatment room, radiology suite, and surgery suite, including an operating room, a surgeon preparation area, an animal preparation area, and a recovery area.[1-3]

Room Construction Features (Macroenvironment)

The term macroenvironment refers to the environment within the room (secondary enclosure) where the dogs are housed. Dog rooms (Figure 2.1) should be constructed with ease of sanitation in mind. The rooms should be equipped with hose stations with ergonomic spray nozzles (Figure 2.2), sloped floors, drain troughs, and floor drains at least 4 in. in diameter to facilitate sanitation and removal of feces. Surface coatings on walls and floors should be made of materials capable of withstanding cleaning by a high-pressure sprayer. Stainless steel wall panels and ceramic blocks hold up better to repeated cleaning than cinder block walls coated with epoxy paint. Flooring types include traditional materials such as ceramic

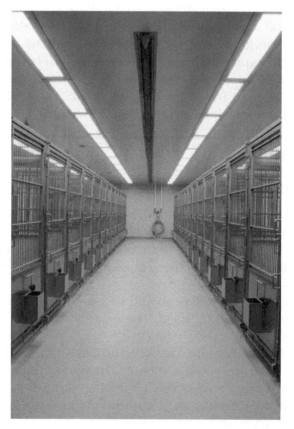

Figure 2.1 Dog kennel room. Note the wide aisle space for easier cleaning and use for dog exercise. Dual hose stations at each end of the room (one pictured) facilitate cleaning in this large kennel. (courtesy of Kevin Johnson, Allentown Incorporated)

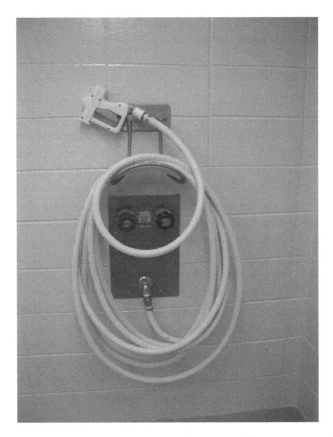

Figure 2.2 An ergonomic spray nozzle is used for spraying down dog kennels. These spray nozzles rotate 360 degrees about the long axis of the hose and reduce wrist fatigue during cleaning.

tiles or troweled on epoxy and newer products such as methylmethacrylate (MMA). MMA offers additional chemical and stain resistance and quicker reuse following installation or repair (within 1 hour). Whatever materials are chosen, the rooms should be maintained in a manner that keeps all surfaces sanitizable and impervious to moisture. Cracks that develop in flooring, walls, or ceilings should be repaired (rebroadcast, sealed, caulked, repainted, etc.) as they occur. Floors should be nonskid, except perhaps under raised-floor kennels and in drain troughs where smoother surfaces facilitate cleaning.

Noise abatement functions can be designed into dog rooms. Acoustical ceiling tiles, wall coverings, and baffles that hang from the ceiling are available in sanitizable materials. Soundproofing doors to dog rooms and entrance airlocks will help lessen the noise in nearby areas of the vivarium.[1-6]

Outdoor Housing

Some facilities maintain dogs in outdoor runs. In general, the use of outdoor housing should be avoided as it adds unnecessary variability into the husbandry program. Dogs housed outdoors are exposed to temperature extremes that do not occur with indoor housing. Even variations in temperature that would not be life threatening or stressful can alter research data by altering the animals' metabolism. In cooler weather, a dog's food intake and metabolism must increase to maintain body temperature. In warmer weather, dogs pant to cool themselves. Although these changes are normal for pet animals, research data can be altered by these changes in metabolism. Dogs housed in outdoor runs must be acclimated to tolerate outdoor conditions.

It is difficult to prevent the exposure of outdoor-housed animals to vermin. Mosquitoes can transmit heartworm disease. Ticks can expose dogs to Rocky Mountain spotted fever and Lyme disease. Fleas (Figure 2.3) and feral rodents can expose dogs to tapeworms. If appropriate perimeter fencing is not maintained, the research animals could be exposed to parvovirus, distemper virus, and even rabies from feral dogs, raccoons, bats, and other species. Many of these diseases can be life threatening, and all have serious consequences to research studies.

If outdoor housing is used, preventive medicine programs should be implemented as compatible with study design. Heartworm prevention, flea and tick control, and vaccination programs should be discussed with the investigator. The products selected and the timing of their use should be coordinated so as not to alter the research data collected.

Note that U.S. Department of Agriculture (USDA) regulations do not permit tethering dogs outside without prior permission from the Animal and Plant Health Inspection Service (APHIS). Dogs housed outdoors must be provided with shelter and shade to protect them from direct sunlight and other environmental conditions such as the wind, rain, or snow.[1-3]

Cage Materials and Design (Microenvironment)

The term microenvironment refers to the environment within the cage or pen (primary enclosure) where the dogs are housed. Dogs are

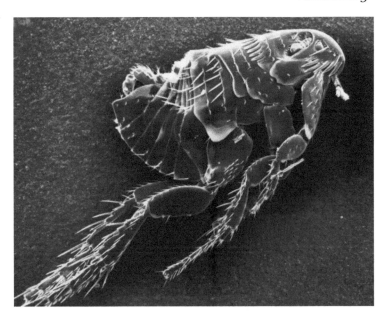

Figure 2.3 *Ctenocephalides felis*, the cat flea, can cause pruritus and dermatitis, and transmits parasites (e.g., tapeworms). They are unlikely to be encountered if indoor housing is used.

typically housed either in cages or runs. All types of housing must be free from sharp edges or points that could injure the animals.

Cages are typically made from stainless steel, as other materials can rust and corrode. Washers, nuts, and small parts used to assemble the cages should also be made from stainless steel, as those made from zinc alloys can be toxic to dogs if ingested.[9–11] Metabolism cages (Figure 2.4) are used for short-duration housing when urine and feces must be collected for analyses. Runs should be constructed of stainless steel, ceramic blocks, or other materials resistant to damage from high-pressure sprayers and from dogs scratching against the walls. Runs can have invertible dividers with solid or gridded panels (Figure 2.5) that permit no or some contact between animals. The dividers can be opened to transfer dogs during cleaning or can be removed to combine runs for group housing of compatible dogs.

For both cages and runs, raised flooring with spaces that allow feces and urine to pass through without entrapping the dogs' footpads is ideal. However, interdigital cysts and footpad lesions may be associated with this type of flooring. Factors to consider are the size and shape of the grid, the type of flooring material, the size and weight of the dogs, and the dampness of the pen floor associated with flushing

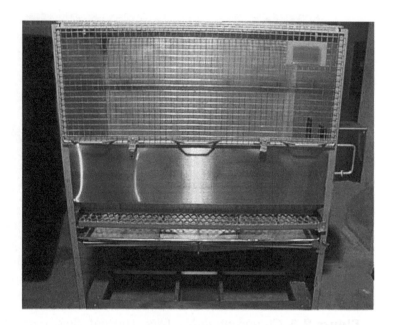

Figure 2.4 Metabolism cages are designed to permit collection of feces and urine during absorption, distribution, metabolism, and excretion (ADME) or pharmacokinetic studies. Often radioisotopes are used to label the test article for easier analyses.

the cages with water. Either slatted flooring (Figure 2.5) or coated metal grid flooring can be used (Figure 2.6). These types of flooring can be heavy and awkward to transport, however. The use of carts facilitates the transportation and sanitization of flooring to and through cage washers (Figure 2.7).

Wood shavings and other bedding materials can be used on the floors of dog runs and can provide excellent housing for dogs, but the purchase of new and disposal of used bedding is costly. Labor involved with cleaning the runs is also increased, as soiled bedding must be scooped out and replaced daily. This is more time consuming than simply hosing feces and urine down the drain. Wood shavings may have a tendency to plug up floor drains, and dogs can ingest them.

Automatic watering systems (Figure 2.8) can be used to decrease the labor involved in caring for dogs. When using automatic watering systems, newly arrived animals should be monitored closely for dehydration, as they may need time to learn how to operate the watering "lixit" valves. Priming the valves by pushing on the lever to start water flow can help new animals learn to operate lixit valves.

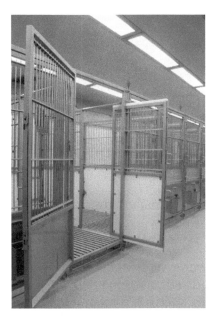

Figure 2.5 A dog kennel with an invertible/removable divider permits no contact (solid panel side down), moderate contact (gridded panel side down), or full contact (remove divider) between dogs. Note also the slatted flooring surface in the kennel. (Courtesy of Kevin Johnson, Allentown Incorporated)

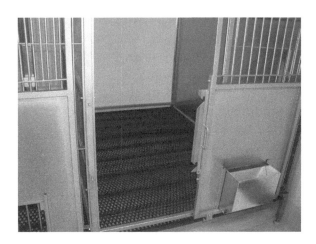

Figure 2.6 Coated metal grid floors are used in this kennel. A J-feeder is seen on the front of the cage and these can be transported to a cage wash for sanitation.

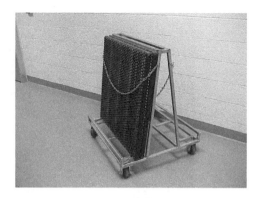

Figure 2.7 Cart transporting cage floors to a cage wash for sanitation in a rack washer.

Automatic watering systems should be checked daily to ensure they are operational. The systems should be flushed periodically according to the manufacturer's recommendations to prevent the buildup of bacteria and biofilms. Water from the system should be analyzed periodically for bacteria, heavy metals, and other contaminants that could affect animal health or research data.

Cage Size Standards

According to USDA animal welfare regulations, the minimum floor space required for a dog is calculated by measuring the dog in inches from the tip of the nose to the base of the tail and adding 6 in. That sum is squared and then divided by 144 to give the minimum square feet of floor space required. The height of the cage must be at least 6 in. higher than the head of the dog when it is in a normal standing position. The space occupied by food bowls, water bowls, and resting boards (Figure 2.8) and other items left on the floor of the cage must be subtracted from the available floor space of the cage. Nursing bitches with litters should be

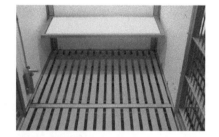

Figure 2.8 Automatic watering "lixit" valve (left) in a kennel with raised resting surface. Unless already trained by the supplier, newly arriving dogs should be trained to use lixit valves to prevent dehydration. Supplemental water bowls can be provided during the training period.

given additional floor space of at least 5% of the bitch's requirement for each pup.

According to the *Guide for the Care and Use of Laboratory Animals*, the floor space required for housing dogs varies by the dogs' weight:

Weight (kg)	Floor space required (ft²)
<15	8.0
Up to 30	12.0
>30	>24.0

Constructing runs or cages with at least twice the minimum required floor space is common practice and provides the opportunity for exercise anytime.

The U.K. minimum floor space requirements for dogs are much larger than in the United States. Larger cages promote species-specific behaviors, provide enrichment and exercise, promote good health, and allow separate areas for sleeping, activity, and excretion.[5]

Environmental Conditions

Light timers should be maintained to ensure an appropriate day-night cycle. Most commonly, 12 hours of light and 12 hours of darkness are used, but a 14 hour light cycle with 10 hours of darkness is also acceptable. If the dog rooms have windows into hallways, using red tinted glass in the windows can help prevent light from the hallway from interfering with the day-night cycle in the room.

Heating, ventilation, and air conditioning (HVAC) systems should maintain the relative humidity between 30% and 70% and the temperature between 64°F and 84°F (18°C to 29°C). Generally relative humidity set points are about 40% to 50% and temperatures are about 68°F to 72°F, which are comfortable ranges for both dogs and personnel. Modern HVAC systems are capable of maintaining room temperatures within 1°F to 2°F (±1°C) of set points and room relative humidity's within 5% to 10% of set points. For most dog rooms, 10 room air changes per hour is appropriate, but increased air flow rates may be needed for high-density housing. If odor is excessive, the airflow should be increased, the room should be cleaned more frequently, and the dogs could be bathed. Air fresheners or scented cleaners should never be used to help alleviate odor problems in dog rooms. Dog room pressurization varies from positive to negative depending on factors such as odor or disease control and HVAC engineering design.

Ideally, environmental conditions should be continuously monitored with appropriate sensors to document environmental conditions. Alarm systems should alert staff if temperature, relative humidity, lighting, or other parameters fall outside set limits. If automated monitoring systems are unavailable, minimum-maximum thermometers should be placed in each room and checked daily. Digital, battery operated units are preferred to the old U-shaped units because the digital units do not contain mercury. The newer, digital units are also capable of monitoring relative humidity and light levels. Portable, handheld devices can be used to spot-check room conditions (Figure 2.9). Temperature and relative humidity sensors should be recalibrated annually to maintain accuracy and correct for drift. Room lighting levels should be monitored for on/off functionality and levels of illumination. Timers or photocells and bulbs should be replaced as needed prior to diminished output. Regular cleaning of light fixture lens covers helps ensure full transmission of available light and proper levels of illumination.[1-6]

animal care

All dogs should be observed at least once daily. Typically, dogs are examined twice daily, at a morning feeding and at an afternoon cage cleaning and health check. Research staff may also provide supplemental observations, especially during studies. Abnormalities should be reported to the veterinary staff for evaluation.

Nutrition and Water

Numerous vendors manufacture laboratory canine diets suitable for research settings. The use of "off-the-shelf" or "supermarket" diets should be avoided, as those brands may change formulations based on changing market prices for ingredients. Although this is acceptable for pet animals, it adds unwanted variability in a research setting.

Both canned and dry foods are available. Dry food is generally preferred for its ease of use and storage, and because it aids the dental health of dogs. The use of J-feeders (Figure 2.6) or bowl holders (Figure 2.14) can help reduce food wastage from spillage. Opened bags of dry diet should be kept in leak-proof containers with tight fitting lids to prevent the entry of insects and other vermin. Open containers of canned food must be refrigerated. Unless otherwise specified by the manufacturer, laboratory canine diets should be used within 6 months of the date of manufacture. According to USDA regulations,

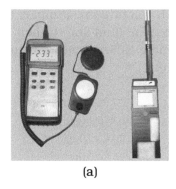

(a)

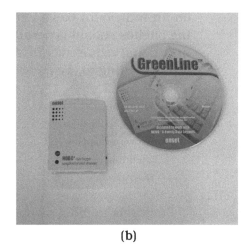

(b)

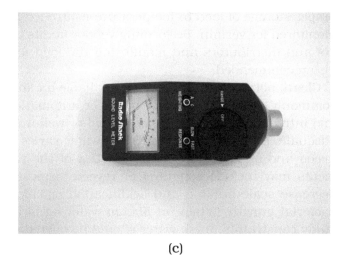

(c)

Figure 2.9 A portable thermohygrometer (a, on right) can be used to measure (spot check) room temperature and relative humidity and a portable light meter (a, on left) can be used to verify illumination levels. Portable programmable digital monitors such as the Hobo data logger (Onset Computer, Bourne, MA) (b) can be used for long-term monitoring of temperature, relative humidity, and light levels and a portable sound meter (c) can be used to monitor noise levels.

only food and bedding that is currently being used may be kept in the animal areas.

Adult dogs can be fed once per day for a few hours. *Ad libitum* feeding may promote obesity in some animals. Limit feeding of dogs on an individual basis can control weight gain. Puppies and nursing bitches should generally be fed *ad libitum* due to their increased nutritional requirements. Approximate caloric requirements for dogs are (according to the *Merck Manual*):

Adult, inactive dogs	50 kcal/kg/day
Adult, active dogs	65 kcal/kg/day
Growing puppies	120 kcal/kg/day
Lactating bitches	200 kcal/kg/day
Heavily worked dogs	450 kcal/kg/day

Programs to monitor the quality of feed received should be implemented. This includes inspecting incoming orders for damage, vermin, and a recent date of manufacture (Figure 2.10) and ensuring proper storage of food in temperature-controlled rooms that are also monitored for vermin. Performing vendor audits of food manufacturers and distributors and monitoring the food for contamination is also recommended.

Clean, potable water should be available *ad libitum*. Water is most commonly provided by water bowls or automatic watering systems and infrequently by bottles. Municipal or well water sources may be adequate, and further treatment of water varies based on research needs and on the local characteristics of the water supply. Treatments may include softening or reverse osmosis of hard water to decrease scale buildup and acidification or chlorination to control bacterial growth. When *ad libitum* watering is not possible due to study constraints, fresh water should be offered several times daily. Provisions for backup water supplies should be established in case the primary water source is interrupted. Daily average water intake for dogs is 20 to 35 ml/kg.

Environmental Enrichment

When compatible with the study design, pair or group housing is the most effective form of environmental enrichment. Dogs are social animals that thrive in group housing situations. Although fighting can occur, it is far less common than with monkeys, mice, or rabbits. For some studies requiring individual measurements of food consumption or other parameters, it is practical to separate group housed dogs into cages during the day and return them to group runs overnight. This allows the best of both worlds for individualized data measurement and group housing enrichment. Kennel dividers

Animal Feed & Bedding Log Form

Product: _____   (lbs) _____

Lot Number	Date Manufactured	Date Received	Quantity Received

Figure 2.10 A feed and bedding receipt log is useful for monitoring product receipt. Products should be inspected for recent date of manufacture, damage, vermin, and quantity.

can be used to provide variable contact between dogs in adjacent runs for added enrichment. Note that USDA regulations require that no more than 12 adult, nonconditioned dogs be housed in the same primary enclosure.

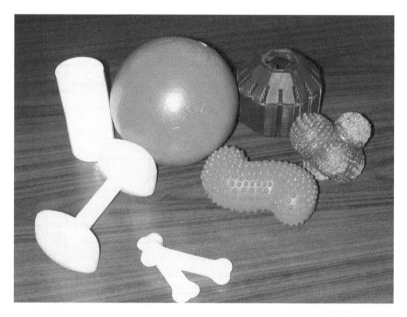

Figure 2.11 A variety of enrichment devices are available for use with lab dogs. Chew toys are commonly used, but all devices should be approved for use by the veterinary and research staff so they do not affect the ongoing research.

A variety of chew toys such as nylabones (Nylabone Products, Neptune City, NJ), gummabones (Nylabone Products, Neptune City, NJ), etc. (Figure 2.11) are available to enrich dogs' environment. These are valuable for all ages of dogs, but especially so for young puppies. Food treats (Figure 2.12) may also be given, but the amounts fed should be specified by the veterinary staff. Food treats should not be given in such quantities as to lessen the amount of the regular diet eaten. Certified chew toys and food treats are available for use in good laboratory practice (GLP) studies.

Finally, positive contact with humans can be especially enriching for both dogs and staff. Caretakers should be allowed adequate time to handle, play with, and walk the animals in order to habituate them to study procedures. Lead training offers good control, provides enrichment and exercise, and decreases staff ergonomic injuries from having to carry dogs. Controlled walks of dogs on leads (Figure 2.13) may be required for research studies (e.g., orthopedic research) or for veterinary purposes and some institutions encourage staff to walk dogs as enrichment. Dogs can be trained to stay in right lateral recumbency for electrocardiogram (EKG) measurement,

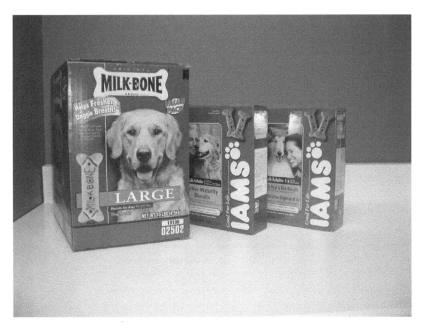

Figure 2.12 Food treats are a source of enrichment for lab dogs. They should be approved for use by the veterinary and research staff and should not be fed to the exclusion of the base diet.

to present their paws for nail trimming, or to open their mouths easily for dosing. Besides being enriching for the animal, time spent in training pays off by improving cooperation and ease of handling during research studies.

Exercise Requirements

According to USDA regulations, individually housed dogs more than 12 weeks old (except bitches with litters) must be provided with a regular opportunity for exercise if they are kept in cages (Figure 2.14) with less than twice the minimum required floor space. The frequency, method, and duration of the opportunity for exercise shall be determined by the attending veterinarian with approval from the Institutional Animal Care and Use Committee (IACUC).

The opportunity for exercise may be provided by allowing access to a run or open area or other similar activities. Forced exercise methods or devices such as swimming, treadmills, or carousel-type devices are unacceptable for meeting the USDA requirement.

Group housed dogs in areas with floor space at least as much as the sum of each individual dog's requirement eliminates the USDA

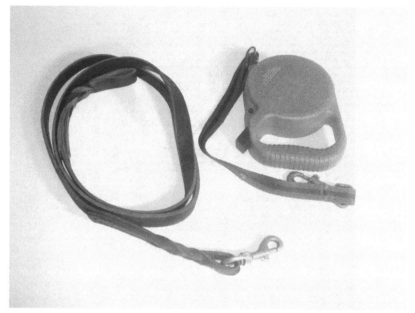

Figure 2.13 Leads are used for control during training of dogs for study use. The increased human contact is enriching and provides exercise. Staff injuries may be decreased when dogs are walked versus carried about the lab.

requirement to provide exercise. Individually housing dogs in areas with more than twice the minimum required floor space also eliminates the requirement for additional exercise.

Constructing runs or cages with at least twice the minimum required floor space is common practice and provides the opportunity for exercise anytime. If resources are available, additional opportunities for exercise may be extended to dogs even when housed in runs or cages with twice the minimum required floor space.

Sanitation

An effective sanitation program is critical for disease prevention and control. USDA regulations require that surfaces in direct contact with dogs be spot cleaned daily (more often if needed) to prevent the accumulation of wastes (food, feces, urine, hair, etc.) and soiling of the animal. Frequent waste removal also provides odor and vermin control and reduces the risk of disease transmission. Cages or runs, feeders, and watering devices (lixits, bowls, bottles, etc.) must be sanitized at least every 2 weeks. Factors affecting overall room

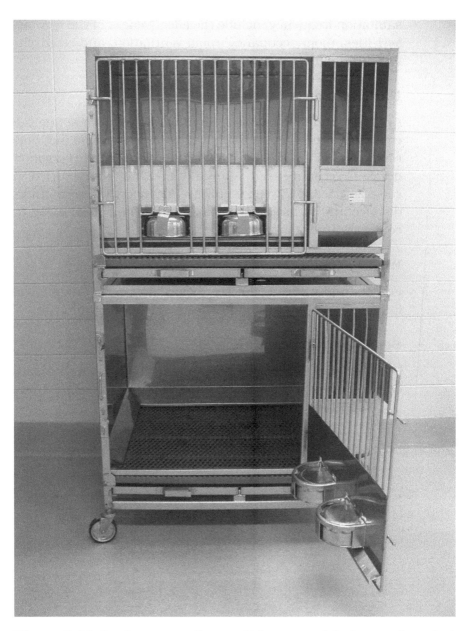

Figure 2.14 Duplex cages (1 over 1's) are used to house dogs, but dogs must be offered exercise periods since the cages have less than 200% of the minimum floor space. Automatic watering can be added to cages instead of the water bowls seen here.

sanitation frequency include the effectiveness of the regular cleaning activities, room occupancy, room ventilation, and research needs. A typical, comprehensive program is as follows:

Daily schedule

Animals should be transferred into clean cages or kennels. Spray the cages or kennels, feeders, and waterers with warm (not hot) water to remove grossly visible waste. Use of a hose with an ergonomic spray nozzle is recommended. Manually brush or scrape dried waste and rinse as needed. Sweep, squeegee, or mop the floor with detergent/disinfectant. If used, chemicals should be rinsed away to prevent contact with dogs.

Weekly schedule

Feeders and watering devices (bowls, bottles) should be transported for sanitation in a mechanical cage washer (Figure 2.15).

Semimonthly schedule

Every 2 weeks, transfer the animals into clean cages. Transport cages, feeders, waterers, and flooring from suspended runs to the

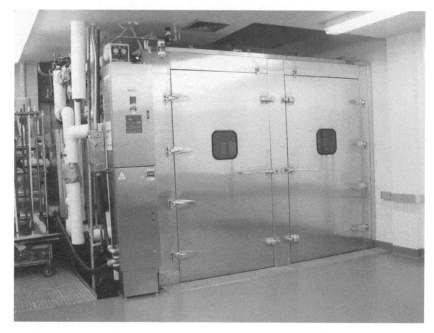

Figure 2.15 A mechanical rack and cage washer is a mainstay for sanitation of caging equipment. Time, temperature (including 180°F final rinse guarantee), and a variety of chemicals are used to ensure sanitation.

cage wash area for sanitation in a mechanical cage washer. Sanitize permanently mounted caging equipment (e.g., runs) in place using portable cleaning equipment and approved chemicals (see below).

Room sanitation schedule

Generally performed monthly to quarterly, remove animals from the room and transport caging equipment (cages, feeders, waterers, removable flooring, dividers, etc.) and supplies (feed and trash barrels, mops, buckets, wringers, squeegees, dust pans, brooms, etc.) to a cage wash area for sanitation in a mechanical cage washer. Sanitize all room and permanently mounted caging equipment (e.g., runs) surfaces. All organic materials such as feces or hair should be removed during the sanitation process. Detergents, disinfectants, and contact time should be capable of destroying vegetative forms of bacteria. Detergents and disinfectants are generally effective, but degreasers and descaling agents (phosphoric or citric acid) may also be needed. Low-pressure sprayers (Figure 2.16) are less damaging to walls and floors than high-pressure sprayers, and low-pressure foamers provide increased contact time. Manual removal by brush or scraper may be needed. All chemicals should be thoroughly rinsed away, and the pens or runs should be dry before returning the animals.

Sanitation quality assurance monitoring

The effectiveness of the sanitization program should be monitored. One method of monitoring is to place replicate organism detection and counting (RODAC) plates (Figure 2.17) on recently sanitized materials and incubate the plates to detect the presence of residual microbial colonies. Another method is to swab recently sanitized materials and insert the swab into a meter that measures light fluorescence as an indicator of the presence of adenosine triphosphate (ATP) from residual organic matter (Figure 2.18). This method requires specialized equipment, but provides instant results, allowing immediate resanitization if needed. Cage washers can be monitored with the use of temperature tapes.

Note: Caution should be maintained to prevent wetting animals during routine cage cleaning. Personnel should wear appropriate personal protective equipment (PPE) such as eye or face protection, gloves, respiratory protection, boots, lab coats, etc., when using chemicals to clean/sanitize dog rooms.

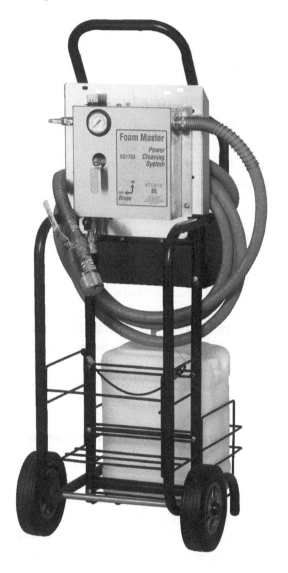

Figure 2.16 A low-pressure metered sprayer/foamer can be used for room sanitation. These sprayers prevent the types of damage seen with high-pressure sprayers. (Courtesy of Jim Walker, Steris Corporation, Mentor, OH)

animal receipt

When a new shipment of dogs arrives at the research facility, receiving staff should evaluate the animals as they are unloaded to ensure

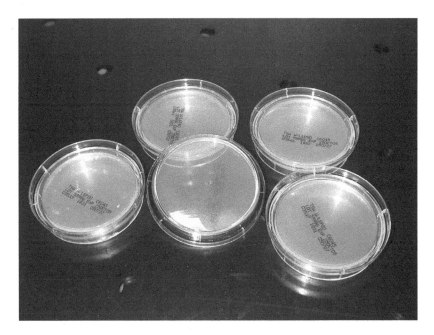

Figure 2.17 RODAC plates are commonly used to monitor for micro-biological growth in facilities. A 48 hour incubation period is required for results.

that the animals received match the animals ordered in breed, age, weight range, sex, and quantity. The animals' tags or tattoos should be matched to the records to verify the animals' identification.

Any health problems should be reported to the veterinary staff immediately. Animals that do not meet purchase order specifications, have antisocial tendencies making them unsafe, or are sick may be rejected. This is especially important for unconditioned, random-source dogs, which may be carrying disease, especially one that is zoonotic. Ideally the animals should be quarantined after arrival before allowing contact with in-house colonies. Diseases that develop secondary to the stress of shipping should be diagnosed and treated without the potential to contaminate in-house colonies. Quarantine, stabilization, and acclimation programs are further described in Chapter 4.

animal identification

According to USDA regulations, all dogs more than 16 weeks of age must be identified by a tag or tattoo. Tags must be made of a durable

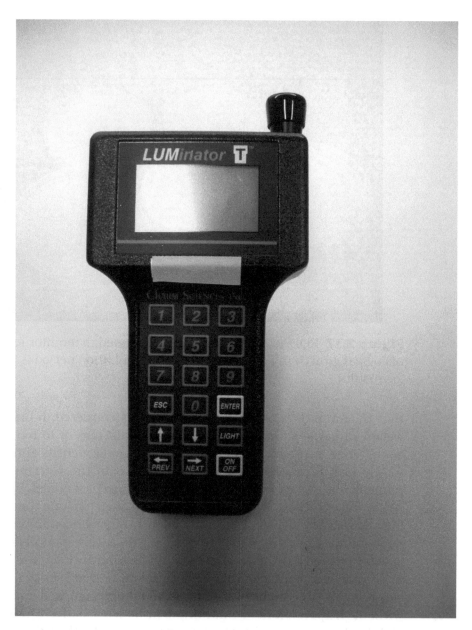

Figure 2.18 Lum-T meters (Charm Sciences, Inc., Malden, MA) are used to monitor for microbiological growth. Swabs are taken from equipment or room surfaces and inserted in a Lum-T meter, which instantly measures the presence of ATP.

material such as brass, bronze, steel, plastic, or aluminum. Tags must be circular and at least 1¼ in. in diameter, or oblong, riveted to a collar, and at least 2 in. long by ¾ in. wide. Each tag must contain the letters "USDA," numbers identifying the state and dealer, exhibitor, or research facility, and numbers identifying the animal. Numbers may not be reused within 5 years. When transferring a dog from one institution to another, the receiving institution can continue to identify the animal with the original tag or tattoo or the receiving institution can affix its own tag or tattoo.

According to the *Guide for the Care and Use of Laboratory Animals*, identification cards (cage cards) should include the source of the animal, names and locations of the responsible investigators, pertinent dates, and the protocol number, when applicable. Microchips implanted subcutaneously in the upper back are being used as a method of identification in some institutions as well. Random-source dogs should be checked for microchip implants upon arrival by scanning the animal with a microchip reader.

transportation

Transportation of dogs to and from as well as within institutions should be performed in a manner that reduces stress, minimizes transport time, and ensures compliance with regulations and standards.[12,13] Key considerations when transporting all animals include the use of proper shipping containers, the availability of food and water, stable environmental conditions, and veterinary care. Health certificates must accompany each dog transported across state lines. The reader should refer to the *Animal Welfare Regulations*, the *Guide for the Care and Use of Laboratory Animals*, and the International Air Transport Association (IATA) series on live animal regulations (the latest is the 32nd edition) for more details about transporting dogs. Described below are the basic standards that apply.

Shipping containers should have the following characteristics: durable, large enough to permit normal postural adjustments, protect the animal from trauma while in transit (i.e., no sharp points or edges), close securely yet permit easy opening during an emergency, provide adequate ventilation, provide protection from drafts, leak proof, and properly labeled.

Food and water must be offered within 4 hours prior to transport. Subsequently water should be provided at least once every 12 hours and food every 12 hours (puppies less than 16 weeks old) to 24 hours (dogs more than 16 weeks old) while in transit. Feeding and watering instructions must accompany shipments. Food and watering devices should be securely attached to the shipping container and should be able to be filled from outside the shipping container.

Environmental conditions should be maintained and monitored during transit to ensure animal well being. The use of environmentally controlled vehicles, capable of providing adequate ventilation and a comfortable temperature is important. Temperature extremes and exposure to inclement weather or direct sunlight should be avoided. Small, portable thermometers can be placed in or among the cages for additional monitoring of ambient temperatures during transit.[14] Deviations from standard conditions should be addressed with transporters.

Observation of dogs in transit is required to be performed at least every 4 hours. General well-being, ventilation, and ambient temperature should be assessed, with appropriate veterinary care provided as needed.

record keeping

Regulations require records of canine acquisition, identification, care, use, and euthanasia/disposal. These records serve as the foundation for good husbandry, veterinary care, and research programs. Records must be retained for 3 years after the completion of an activity (e.g., study use). Dog tags should be retained for at least 1 year. Refer to the *Animal Welfare Regulations* for additional details on records. Described below are records commonly used in research facilities.

Husbandry Records

Husbandry records or room activity logs (Figure 2.19) are used to document the performance of regular husbandry tasks. These may include arrival records, daily health checks, the provision of feed and water, cage cleaning or changing, and room temperature and humidity checks. Technicians performing the tasks should initial, date, and indicate the time activities are performed.

Census records are used to track the numbers of animals in house over the course of the year on a regular basis (e.g., daily or weekly). The information is used to bill per diems, to determine room and facility occupancy, to assess workload, and to provide information for USDA annual reports.

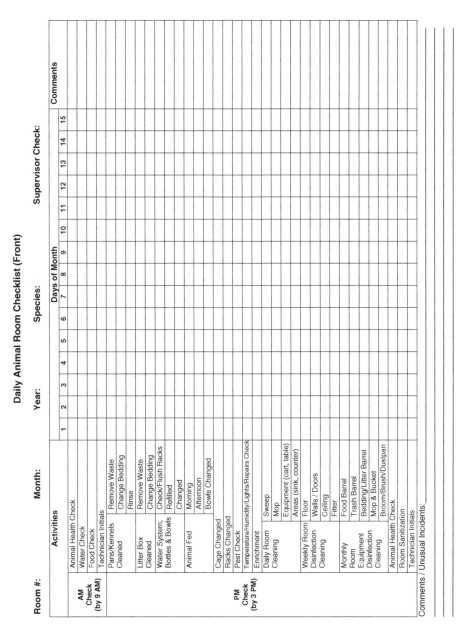

Figure 2.19 A multispecies room activity log is commonly used to document completion of routine husbandry activities. Tasks should be marked off (checkmark or initials) when completed.

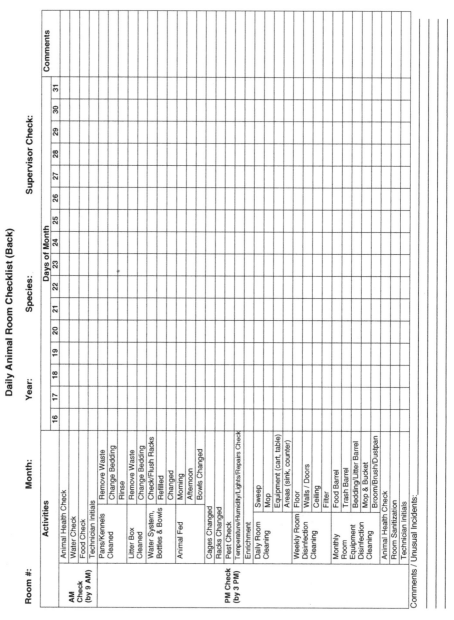

Figure 2.19 (continued)

Medical records are used to document the care animals receive. These include the results of health exams, clinical findings, diagnostic tests and procedures, prophylactic vaccinations and anthelmintic treatments, anesthesia, surgical and perioperative records, veterinary treatments, research interventions, and necropsy findings. Consulting with the attending veterinarian is critical to developing a comprehensive medical records program. Refer to the American College of Laboratory Animal Medicine (ACLAM) *Public Statements: Medical Records for Animals Used for Research, Teaching and Testing* for additional details on medical records.[15]

references

1. Hessler, J.R. and Moreland, A.F., Design and management of animal facilities, in *Laboratory Animal Medicine*, Fox, J.G., Cohen, B.J., and Loew, F.M., eds., Academic Press, San Diego, 1984, chap. 20.

2. Hessler, J.R. and Leary, S.L., Design and management of animal facilities, in *Laboratory Animal Medicine*, 2nd ed., Fox, J.G., Anderson, L.C., Loew, F.M., and Quimby, F.W., eds., Academic Press, San Diego, 2002, chap. 21.

3. Committee on the Care and Use of Laboratory Animals of the Institute for Laboratory Animal Resources, *Guide for the Care and Use of Laboratory Animals*, 7th ed., National Academy Press, Washington, DC, 1996, chap. 2.

4. Code of Federal Regulations, Title 9, Parts 1, 2, and 3 (Docket 89-130), *Federal Register*, vol. 54, no. 168, August 31, 1989, and 9 CFR Part 3 (Docket 90-218), *Federal Register*, vol. 56, no. 32, February 15, 1991.

5. Joint Working Group on Refinement, Refining dog husbandry and care, *Lab. Anim.*, 38 (suppl. 1), 1, 2004.

6. Committee on Dogs of the Institute for Laboratory Animal Resources, *Laboratory Animal Management: Dogs*, National Academy Press, Washington, DC, 1994.

7. Bonagura, J.D., *Kirk's Veterinary Therapy XIII: Small Animal Practice*, WB Saunders, Philadelphia, 2000.

8. Kahn, C.M. and Line, S., eds. *The Merck Veterinary Manual*, 9th ed., Merck & Co., Whitehouse Station, NJ, 2005.

9. Volmer, P.A., Roberts, J., and Meerdink, G.L., Anuric renal failure associated with zinc toxicosis in a dog, *Vet. Hum. Toxicol.*, 46, 276, 2004.

10. Hammond, G.M., Loewen, M.E., and Blakely, B.R., Diagnosis and treatment of zinc poisoning in a dog, *Vet. Hum. Toxicol.*, 46, 272, 2004.

11. Robinette, C.L., Toxicology of selected pesticides, drugs, and chemicals. Zinc, *Vet. Clin. North Am. Small Anim. Pract.*, 20, 539, 1990.

12. Guidelines for the care of laboratory animals in transit, Laboratory Animal Breeders Association of Great Britain Limited (LABA) and Laboratory Animal Science Association (LASA), Association of the British Pharmaceutical Industry (ABPI), British Laboratory Animal Veterinary Association (BLAVA), Institute of Animal Technology (IAT), Ministry of Agriculture, Fisheries & Food (MAFF), Universities Federation for Animal Welfare (UFAW), and Animals (Scientific Procedures) Inspectorate, *Lab. Anim.*, 27, 93, 1993.

13. International Air Transport Association, *Live Animal Regulations*, 32nd ed., International Air Transport Association, Montreal, Quebec, Canada, 2005.

14. Mean, J., Mice on the move, in Report of the 2004 RSPCA/UFAW rodent welfare group meeting.

15. Medical Records Committee, American College of Laboratory Animal Medicine, *Public Statements: Medical Records for Animals Used for Research, Teaching and Testing*, American College of Laboratory Animal Medicine, Chester, NH, 2004.

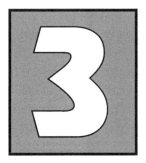

management

regulatory agencies and compliance

Dogs are a very high profile species in the eyes of regulatory agencies. The original Laboratory Animal Welfare Act (Public Law 89-544) was passed in 1966 after a missing pet Dalmatian was used in a medical experiment in a New York hospital. Although the original intent of the act was to curb pet theft, it was amended in 1970, 1976, 1985, and 1990 to include standards for laboratory animal care. Summarized below are the regulatory and accrediting agencies that may impact the use of dogs in research.

U.S. Department of Agriculture

The U.S. Department of Agriculture (USDA) is charged by the Animal Welfare Act with promulgating and enforcing standards of animal care. The Animal and Plant Health Inspection Service (APHIS), Animal Care is headquartered in Maryland with regional offices in North Carolina and Colorado. Research facilities using dogs are required to register with the USDA, and dealers of dogs must be licensed by Animal Care. Veterinary medical officers and animal care inspectors perform unannounced inspections of research facilities, dealers, zoos, and exhibitors using dogs and other species.

The specific standards of care are listed in the *Code of Federal Regulations*, Title 9—Animals and Animal Products. They can be viewed on the USDA's publication site at http://www.aphis.usda.gov/ac/publications.html. Animal Care also makes available their policy manual, which is used to guide veterinary medical officers and animal care inspectors in how to interpret the regulations. The policy manual may be viewed at http://www.aphis.usda.gov/ac/polmanpdf.html.

The regulations provide strict engineering standards for dog housing and their use in research. There are provisions for minimum cage sizes, the exercise of dogs, and requirements for providing veterinary care. There are strict identification and record keeping requirements, as well as rules for sanitation of primary enclosures. Failure to adhere to the regulations can lead to regulatory citations, fines, and loss of licensure or registration. To maintain registration, research facilities must file an annual report by December 1 of each year with Animal Care listing the number of dogs used in research, teaching, and testing.

Public Health Service, National Institutes of Health, and Office for Laboratory Animal Welfare

The Health Research Extension Act of 1985 (Public Law 99-158) directed the Secretary of Health and Human Services to establish guidelines for the proper care of animals used in biomedical and behavioral research. As a result, the Public Health Service (PHS) Policy on Humane Care and Use of Laboratory Animals was created. All institutions receiving grants from the PHS must abide by this policy. The policy is administered through the National Institutes of Health (NIH) Office for Laboratory Animal Welfare.

Public Health Service policy requires all institutions receiving financial support from the PHS for animal research to file an animal welfare assurance statement with the Office for Laboratory Animal Welfare (OLAW). This legally binding document outlines how institutions will meet PHS requirements for animal care of all vertebrate species including dogs. PHS policy requires that institutions maintain the standards for animal care listed in the *Guide for the Care and Use of Laboratory Animals* published by the Institute for Laboratory Animal Resources. To maintain their assurance, institutions must also file annual reports with OLAW listing any changes in the program of care for all vertebrate animals.

Helpful information on the PHS policy, how to file an assurance statement, how to prepare an annual report, and other information can be found on OLAW's website at http://grants.nih.gov/grants/olaw/olaw.htm. Failure to comply with PHS policy can result in loss of PHS financial support.

U.S. Food and Drug Administration and U.S. Environmental Protection Agency Good Laboratory Practice Regulations

Good laboratory practice (GLP) regulations are published in the *Code of Federal Regulations*, Title 21—Food and Drugs. They are intended to protect the quality of data submitted to gain U.S. Food and Drug Administration (FDA) approval of pharmaceuticals and medical devices and to gain U.S. Environmental Protection Agency (EPA) approval of pesticides and other chemicals. Some specific regulations relate to the care of laboratory animals, including dogs. The regulations require facilities to develop and follow standard operating procedures (SOPs) for performing studies and to set up a quality assurance unit to monitor how well the SOPs are followed. FDA auditors enforce the GLPs through unannounced inspections. Failure to comply can result in regulatory citations and the inability to use study results to gain agency approval of products.

The Association for Assessment and Accreditation of Laboratory Animal Care International

The Association for Assessment and Accreditation of Laboratory Animal Care (AAALAC) International is a private, nonprofit agency that accredits animal care and use programs. AAALAC is governed by a board of directors made up of representatives from more than 30 organizations, including the American Association for Laboratory Animal Science, the American Medical Association, and the American Veterinary Medical Association. Accreditation is voluntary and demonstrates commitment to appropriate animal care and compliance with the laws and regulations governing animal research.

Accreditation is earned by passing an extensive peer review process, including evaluation of a written description of the institution's animal care program as well as a formal site visit by members of AAALAC's Council on Accreditation and ad hoc consultants. Site visits are conducted every 3 years. AAALAC does not promulgate its own standards of animal care, but ensures compliance with regulatory agency guidelines and current professional standards. The main reference used by AAALAC is the *Guide for the Care and Use of Laboratory Animals*. More information about AAALAC accreditation can be found at http://www.aaalac.org.

State and local agencies

Some states and local municipalities also regulate animal research involving dogs. These agencies may send their inspectors to review institutions' animal care programs.

institutional animal care and use committee

USDA regulations, PHS policy, and the *Guide for the Care and Use of Laboratory Animals* all require Institutional Animal Care and Use Committees (IACUCs) to oversee each institution's program of animal care. These committees are responsible for reviewing complete descriptions of animal activities and approving those activities in advance of any procedures being performed. **No use of dogs in teaching, education, or research may take place in the United States without prior approval from the local IACUC.**

An IACUC must include members with diverse backgrounds to give balance and perspective to their collective judgment. Both USDA's regulations and PHS policy require the IACUC to have a veterinarian with training or experience caring for laboratory animals. Both require a community member not affiliated with the institution to represent the interests of the general public. USDA regulations require a chairperson and PHS policy requires both a scientist and a nonscientist be committee members. The chief executive officer of the institution must appoint IACUC members. Responsibilities of the IACUC include:

- Perform a semiannual review of the research facility's program for humane care and use of animals and an inspection of the institution's animal facilities, including the animal study areas.

- Prepare reports of the semiannual inspections and program reviews and submit them to the Institutional Official. The report should describe areas of compliance and noncompliance. For any deficiencies found while inspecting the facilities or reviewing the program, the IACUC must set a timely and specific plan for correcting the problem and follow up to ensure the deficiency is corrected.

- Review and investigate concerns regarding proper care and use of animals.

- Make recommendations to the Institutional Official regarding the research facilities and program for care and use of animals.

- Review proposed activities (protocols) for animal use and significant changes to approved animal use activities. Protocols may be approved, have approval withheld, or be approved following modification. Protocols must be approved by the IACUC before they can begin.
- Suspend activities using animals.
- Ensure that the investigator has considered alternatives to procedures that may cause more than momentary pain or distress and that the research is not duplicative of other research.
- Ensure that the animals are properly housed, fed, watered, maintained, and cared for. This includes ensuring proper veterinary care.
- Ensure that anesthesia, surgery, and perioperative care are performed appropriately.
- Ensure that pain, discomfort, and distress are minimized or avoided in procedures used on animals.
- Ensure that proper methods of euthanasia of animals are used.
- Ensure that personnel performing procedures on animals and providing care to animals are properly trained.

Overall, it is the role of the IACUC to balance the ethical cost of performing any animal activity; that is, the IACUC must determine whether the potential benefit from performing a study outweighs any potential pain or distress that could be experienced by the animals and any potential loss of animal life. This tremendous power and overriding authority invested in the IACUC must be taken seriously. IACUCs are required to document their actions, and regulatory and accrediting agencies review this documentation carefully to ensure that IACUCs fulfill their responsibilities.[1,2]

occupational health and safety

Public Health Service policy and the *Guide for the Care and Use of Laboratory Animals* require an occupational health and safety program for all individuals working with laboratory animals, including dogs. The program should involve an assessment of the risks relative to the type of work performed. The type of safety program should be tailored to mitigate the risks involved. In 1997 the National Research Council published comprehensive guidance on this topic in *Occupational Health and Safety in the Care of Research Animals*.

The main hazards associated with laboratory dogs are physical injuries such as bites or scratches and allergies. Most purpose-bred laboratory canines are docile and easier to work with than small breed, pet animals. Breeders of research dogs work hard to socialize their animals so that they readily tolerate handling by people. Random-source animals are more likely to have socialization problems. Inexperienced employees should receive training in canine behavior, how to recognize aggression in individual dogs, and how to properly restrain fractious animals. The use of poorly socialized or aggressive animals should be avoided, especially in long-term studies. All employees working with laboratory canines should be offered a tetanus vaccination.

Allergies to dogs are a potentially serious occupational health and safety issue. Discussion of allergies with personnel who work with animals should be a part of the preemployment physical examination for people seeking employment in animal research facilities. Employees who develop symptoms such as nasal discharge or sneezing after working with dogs should report these symptoms to their supervisor and seek advice from an occupational health professional.

Institutions using random-source dogs should verify the rabies vaccination status of all dogs acquired from their suppliers. Preferentially, suppliers should be required to vaccinate dogs against rabies. Otherwise, institutions should vaccinate dogs upon arrival. Workers at risk should consider a preexposure vaccination.

The common forms of personal protective equipment used when handling laboratory dogs include lab coats or uniforms, shoe covers, and examination gloves. Boots are usually worn when hosing down runs. Caps, masks, or respirators, safety shoes, and safety glasses or face shields may be used depending on the type of work involved.[3]

zoonoses

Zoonotic diseases are diseases transmitted from animals to man. Zoonotic diseases from handling purpose-bred laboratory dogs are rare. These animals are not exposed to the range of disease organisms associated with animals allowed to roam freely outdoors. Random-source dogs are more likely to have been exposed to zoonotic disease agents, but these animals are typically held for a conditioning period to detect and treat disease before they are used experimentally. Unless the dogs are inoculated experimentally with hazardous agents, the chance of acquiring a zoonotic disease from exposure to laboratory canines is low. However, because the consequences are potentially severe, appropriate precautionary measures should still be used when handling these animals.[4-6] Important zoonotic diseases of dogs are discussed below.

Rabies

Rabies is a rare, but extremely serious viral disease of mammals. Human exposure to rabies virus is normally fatal unless prophylactic treatment is provided immediately after an exposure, before symptoms develop. The virus is transmitted via the saliva through the bite of a rabid animal. Airborne transmission may occur from mucous membrane exposure to the urine of infected bats.

Although it is almost impossible for a purpose-bred dog to be exposed to a rabid animal, it would be possible for a stray dog to be exposed before being captured by a pound. Hence the possibility of contracting rabies from working with random-source laboratory canines is higher than that from working with purpose-bred animals. Effective vaccines are available and are often part of the conditioning program for laboratory dogs. Vaccines are also available to protect humans and are part of the occupational health and safety programs of many institutions where dogs are used. The occupational health program must address employee exposure to dog saliva by bites and wounds. Typically a dog is observed for clinical signs of rabies for a 10 day period following human exposure by a bite or scratch.[4-6]

Scabies

Dogs can be infested with the mange mite, *Sarcoptes scabei*. This mite causes hair loss and intense pruritus in infected dogs. Skin scrapings are used to diagnose the disease, but a negative scraping does not rule out scabies. Various medications such as oral ivermectin or milbemycin can be used to kill the mites.

When humans have direct contact with infected dogs, the mite can burrow into the human's skin. This results in pimples or rashes with intense itching. Although the mites contracted from dogs cannot reproduce in people and the infestation will cure itself, medication may be used to shorten the course of the disease and lessen the discomfort. Humans can be carriers of a similar scabies mite that can reproduce in humans and requires treatment to eliminate.[4-6]

Intestinal Helminthes

Various intestinal helminthes in dogs can cause disease in humans. Hookworm (*Ancylostoma* sp.) and roundworm (*Toxocara* sp.) larvae can enter humans and migrate through the body causing damage. Entry occurs through larval penetration of the skin or by ingestion of soil or unwashed, raw vegetables contaminated with infective eggs, which hatch and migrate through the intestinal wall into the body. Depending on where the larvae migrate, they can cause skin disease, neurological problems from damage to the brain or spinal cord, and even blindness from entering the eye. Tapeworms (*Echinococcus* sp. and *Dipylidium caninum*) can also infect people. Periodic testing and treatment of dogs for intestinal parasites, maintaining good sanitation of dog housing areas, and employee hand washing are excellent methods of prevention.[4-6]

Giardiasis

Giardia sp. are protozoa that cause intestinal disease in a wide variety of animals, including dogs and humans. Diarrhea is the most common clinical sign. Transmission is by a fecal-oral route when a dog carrying giardia sheds infective cysts with their feces. Another dog sniffs the contaminated feces and infective cysts are inadvertently "ingested." Diagnosis is by microscopic examination of fecal samples, looking for giardial cysts. The use of exam gloves and hand washing are the best preventive measures. Prohibition of eating, drinking, smoking, or application of cosmetics within the animal facility are other standard preventive measures.[4-6]

Infections Resulting from Bite Wounds

Bite wound infections generally occur from bites to the hands and arms of animal caretakers or other personnel having increased contact with dogs. Infections are caused by normal aerobic and anaerobic flora of the oral cavity of the dog, often acting in concert, which complicates treatment. Bacteria may include *Pasteurella multocida*, *Staphylococcus* sp., *Escherichia coli*, *Mycoplasma* sp., *Enterobacter aerogenes*, *Moraxella* sp., *Capnocytophaga canimorus*, and others. Localized and systemic infections may result and personnel should obtain prompt medical attention. Unsocial, aggressive, or fearful dogs that are at increased risk of biting personnel should not be kept.[7-10]

human-animal bond

The human-animal bond, or the relationship between people and animals, is an important consideration in research facilities. USDA regulations detail core programmatic requirements that include "adequate veterinary care," "appropriately qualified and trained personnel," "daily observation of all animals to assess their health and well-being," and "psychological well-being." Scientists have long recognized that humane care of animals is an important factor contributing to the success and advancement of their research.[11] Animal facility management emphasizes compassion and caring as much as education, training, and experience during recruitment of animal care staff. Pet ownership is common among animal care and research staff. Dogs' strong social tendencies coupled with their playful, docile nature increase the likelihood of bonding. In light of these factors, some bonding with dogs and other higher laboratory species is inevitable, particularly for those having the greatest contact, such as animal caretakers and research technicians. Science and research personnel can be affected, both positively and negatively, by the human-animal bond.[12]

Organizations have strong scientific as well as moral, ethical, and legal obligations to address the human-animal bond. Benefits to science, personnel, and animals seem clear, as does the risk of not doing so.[13-17] Formal recognition of the human-animal bond on an institutional level is needed to address the issue most effectively and has been done by some institutions.[18] Broad staff participation and support of senior institutional officials is essential in developing a program that recognizes and manages the human-animal bond to maximize benefits and minimize any negative consequences to science, animals, and staff. Programs should involve research and animal caretaker staff, veterinarians, the IACUC, and the Institutional Official. Equally important is documenting the methods and results achieved. For further reading on this subject, an excellent reference is the *ILAR Journal*, Implications of Human-Animal Interactions and Bonds in the Laboratory (43, 1, 2002).

references

1. Code of Federal Regulations, Title 9, Parts 1, 2, and 3 (Docket 89-130), *Federal Register*, vol. 54, no. 168, August 31, 1989, and 9 CFR Part 3 (Docket 90-218), *Federal Register*, vol. 56, no. 32, February 15, 1991.

2. Committee on the Care and Use of Laboratory Animals of the Institute for Laboratory Animal Resources, *Guide for the Care and Use of Laboratory Animals*, 7th ed., National Academy Press, Washington, DC, 1996, chap. 2.

3. Committee on Occupational Safety and Health in Research Animal Facilities of the Institute of Laboratory Animal Resources, *Occupational Health and Safety in the Care and Use of Research Animals*, National Academy Press, Washington, DC, 1997.

4. Kahn, C.M. and Line, S., eds., *The Merck Veterinary Manual*, 9th ed., Merck & Co., Whitehouse Station, NJ, 2005.

5. Greene, C.E., ed., *Clinical Microbiology and Infectious Diseases of the Dog and Cat*, W.B. Saunders, Philadelphia, 1984.

6. Dysko, R.C., Nemzek, J.A., Levin, S.I., DeMarco, G.J., and Moalli, M.R., Biology and diseases of dogs, in *Laboratory Animal Medicine*, 2nd ed., Fox, J.G., Anderson, L.C., Loew, F.M., and Quimby, F.W., eds., Academic Press, San Diego, 2002, chap. 11.

7. August, J.R., Dog and cat bites. *J. Am. Vet. Med. Assoc.*, 193, 1394, 1988.

8. Talan, D.A., Citron, D.M., Abrahamian, F.M., Moran, G.J., and Goldstein, E.J.C., Bacteriologic analysis of infected dog and cat bites. *N. Engl. J. Med.*, 340, 85, 1999.

9. Drobatz, K.J. and Smith, G., Evaluation of risk factors for bite wounds inflicted on caregivers by dogs and cats in a veterinary teaching hospital, *J. Am. Vet. Med. Assoc.*, 223, 312, 2003.

10. Job, L., Horman, J.T., Grigor, J.K., and Israel, E., Dysgonic fermenter-2: a clinico-epidemiologic review. *J. Emerg. Med.*, 7, 185, 1989.

11. Weed, J.L. and Raber, J.M., Balancing animal research with animal well-being: establishment of goals and harmonization of approaches, *ILAR J.*, 46, 118, 2005.

12. Wolfe, T.L., Introduction: Implications of the human-animal interactions and bonds in the laboratory, *ILAR J.*, 43, 1, 2002.

13. Bayne, K., Development of the human-research animal bond and its impact on animal well-being, *ILAR J.*, 43, 4, 2002.

14. Chang, F.T. and Hart, L.A., Human-animal bonds in the laboratory: how animal behavior affects the perspectives of caregivers, *ILAR J.*, 43, 10, 2002.

15. Davis, H., Prediction and preparation: Pavlovian implications of research animals discriminating among humans, *ILAR J.*, 43, 19, 2002.

16. Herzog, H., Ethical aspects of relationships between humans and research animals, *ILAR J.*, 43, 27, 2002.

17. Russow, L.M., Ethical implications of the human-animal bond in the laboratory, *ILAR J.*, 43, 33, 2002.

18. Iliff, S.A., An additional "R": remembering the animals, *ILAR J.*, 43, 38, 2002.

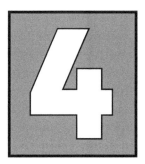

veterinary care

---

preventive health program

A key component of an institution's veterinary care program is a sound preventive health program. Institution's should develop a program that best fits their unique needs, including specific research goals and veterinary resources (personnel, equipment, and supplies). A veterinarian knowledgeable in providing veterinary care for dogs should develop and oversee preventive health programs. Elements of a program are described below and include identifying reliable sources of healthy research dogs and developing appropriate quarantine, stabilization, acclimation, and colony separation programs.

Sources

Dogs can be obtained from a variety of sources, but are generally classified into two types: purpose-bred and random-source dogs. As the name implies, purpose-bred dogs are bred solely for use in research and are obtained from class "A" licensees (i.e., breeders), while random-source dogs may be bred for multiple uses. Animals such as retired racing dogs, strays, etc., are obtained from class "B" licensees (i.e., dealers).

Important factors in selecting an appropriate dog source include the institutional research goals, the institution's health standards for dogs, the veterinary care program of the suppliers, and the institution's budget. For example, when research objectives require long-term studies, dog selection may differ significantly from institutions with short-term research objectives. In the former case, healthier dogs with a known medical history are preferred versus the latter case in which dogs with incomplete medical histories may be acceptable.

Institutional health standards for dogs can vary from very high, requiring the dogs to be free of common pathogens and to have been vaccinated and treated prophylactically for endo- and ectoparasites prior to arrival, to lower standards where dogs may have received limited prior vaccinations and parasite treatments. Institutional health standards may be defined as part of the facility's bioexclusion list of excluded pathogens for all species of animals, including dogs.

Class A dealers (breeders) customarily develop their veterinary care programs to meet research needs. They typically have complete programs of veterinary care at their production sites. Class B dealers' programs can vary widely from high to minimal standards. Overall, purpose-bred dogs should be free of common canine pathogens such as viruses and parasites. Purpose-bred dogs are usually more expensive than random-source dogs. An excellent resource for identifying specific sources of dogs is the buyers guide published annually by *Lab Animal* magazine (Nature Publishing Group, New York).

Quarantine, Stabilization, and Acclimation

The quarantine, stabilization, and acclimation (QSA) program covers practices and procedures from the initial receipt of a group of dogs until they are released for use in research. During this period of time, dogs are allowed to recover from shipping stress, acclimate to their new environment and diet, and have their health status evaluated. Personnel access should be limited to animal care personnel, research should be disallowed, and sample collections should be limited to those samples necessary for health evaluation.

The rigor and duration of the QSA program should also consider the quality of dogs selected and the vendor's transportation procedures. Dogs obtained from approved vendors with acceptable health profiles may require a short acclimation and stabilization period rather than a true quarantine. Monitoring of vendors, including examining health reports of incoming animals, monitoring vendor health surveillance reports, and performing site inspections of approved vendors are important oversight mechanisms. The method of transport should not expose animals to pathogens or environmental stress. QSA periods of 1 to 2 weeks are typical for animals from known sources, while longer periods are needed for animals obtained from random-source dealers with uncertain health status.

Colony Separation

Colony separation refers to separation of animals by health status, vendor source, and type or breed. The need for separation is determined largely by research needs, housing space, vendor health profiles, and current health status of resident colonies. Institutions should provide for housing animals during QSA, after release from QSA in general housing, in study-specific housing if needed, and in separate housing areas for ill or potentially infectious animals. Species separation should be maintained, and animals can be further separated by vendor and type (purpose bred versus random source). In general, during the QSA period, incoming dogs obtained from approved vendors can be housed in colony rooms with other dogs of similar health status and vendor origin.

clinical management

Basic Veterinary Supplies

A variety of basic veterinary supplies are important to have available in order to perform routine veterinary care of dogs. Listed below are some of the items one should maintain in or near the treatment/examination room. Other equipment and supplies may be indicated as well.

- A stethoscope (Figure 4.1)
- Rectal thermometer (digital preferred) and plastic sleeves (Figure 4.1)
- Water-soluble lubricating jelly
- Examination gloves and a lab coat
- Scale to weigh the animal
- An examination table with or without a nonslip mat
- Penlight and ophthalmoscope (Figure 4.2)
- Blood collection tubes with an additive such as ethylenediaminetetraacetic acid (EDTA) (purple top) for collection of whole blood or without additives for collection of serum (red top)
- Microhematocrit tubes
- Antiseptics such as povidone-iodine solution, chlorhexidine, or alcohol
- Nail clippers and hemostatic agents (Figure 4.3)

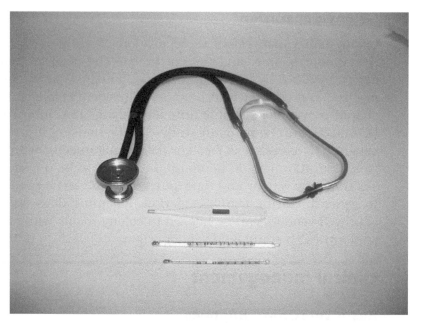

Figure 4.1 Basic tools of the trade: a stethoscope, a digital thermometer, and two sizes of mercury thermometers.

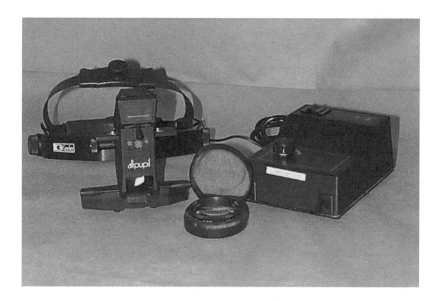

Figure 4.2 An indirect ophthalmoscope is used to perform eye examinations.

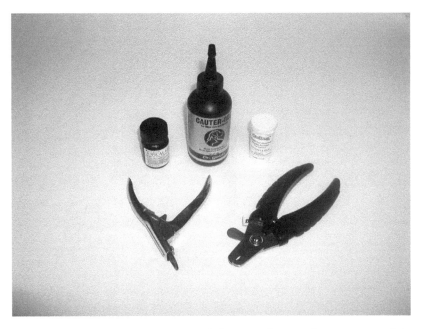

Figure 4.3 Nail clippers are used for regular nail trimming. Hemostatic agents are needed when a toenail bleeds if it is clipped too short or is torn during activity.

- Disposable syringes ranging in size from 1 to 50 ml (luer lock and catheter tip)
- Disposable needles ranging from 18 to 27 gauge of varying lengths from 5/8 in. to 1½ in.
- Disposable indwelling catheters ranging from 18 to 24 gauge and 2 in. to 4 in. long
- Hair clippers with a number 40 blade and a high efficiency particulate air (HEPA) filtered vacuum
- Bandaging materials such as nonstick pads, roll or pad gauze, cotton balls, adhesive tape (e.g., Elastikon; Johnson & Johnson, New Brunswick, NJ), self-adherent wraps (e.g., Vetrap; 3M, St. Paul, MN), and padding
- Bandage scissors
- Laryngoscope
- Muzzle
- Otoscope
- Oral and vaginal speculums

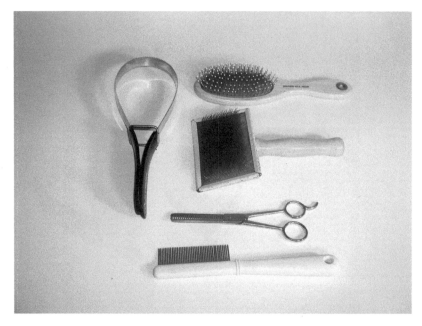

Figure 4.4 Grooming equipment (brushes, combs, and scissors) is used to maintain a dog's hair coat. Grooming provides tactile stimulation to dogs and can be part of a facility's socialization and enrichment program.

- Sterile fluids, such as 0.9% saline or lactated Ringers and intravenous administration sets (standard and micro-drip sets)
- Sterile bacterial culture swabs and media
- Sterile specimen containers for collection of urine samples
- Specimen container for collection of fecal samples
- Circulating hot water heating pad
- Grooming equipment (Figure 4.4)
- Sterile pack with assortment of surgical instruments such as scalpel holder, tissue forceps, tissue scissors, gauze, suture needle holders, suture scissors, tissue staples, and stapler
- Sterile absorbable and nonabsorbable suture packs of varying gauges ranging from 0-0 to 5-0
- Oral feeding tubes (Figure 4.5)
- Dental machine and hand instruments such as hand scalers, probes, curettes, and a mirror (Figure 4.6)

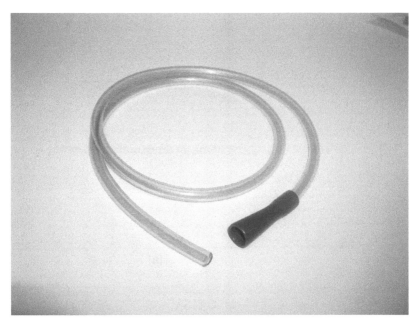

Figure 4.5 A stomach tube is used for feeding, dosing animals with liquid formulations, or to evacuate the stomach contents during emergency procedures.

The Physical Examination

A thorough physical examination is the cornerstone of adequate veterinary care of dogs. It should be performed on all dogs upon arrival at the facility to verify conformation with the purchase order, facility, or study-related health standards and it serves as a baseline for future comparison. Subsequent physical examinations should be performed based on the development of clinical abnormalities, as part of routine prophylactic veterinary care programs (semiannual to annual examinations, reuse following rest/study withdrawal periods, etc.), as part of study protocols, and as part of pet adoption programs. Records of the examination (Figure 4.7) should be maintained as part of the individual animal's medical record, including the results of all diagnostic testing performed. Physical examinations should always be done systematically, so that no areas are overlooked.

Examination rooms proximal in location to housing/study areas offer operational advantages and may reduce stress on the dogs from transportation. Physical examinations should be performed in quiet, well-lighted examination rooms, preferably with an assistant

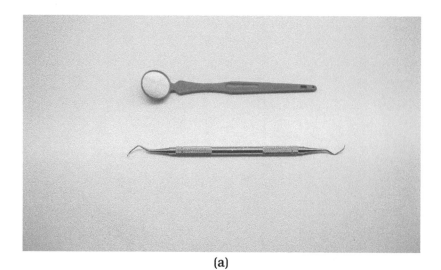

(a)

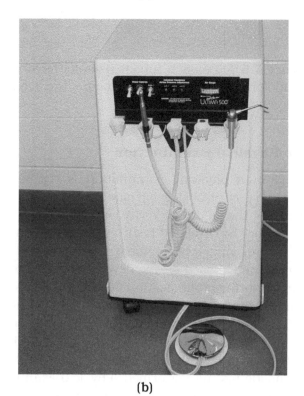

(b)

Figure 4.6 (a) Manual dental equipment is used to examine and hand clean teeth. (b) Dogs kept long-term will benefit from dental care programs where dental units with ultrasonic scalers are used to clean teeth with more extensive calculus buildup.

Clinical Examination Record

Protocol Number: _____ Principle Investigator:_____ Extension:_____

Animal ID: _____Date: _____Species: _____

Breed: _____Identifying Markings: _____

Temperature (°F): _____ Respiration Rate _____Heart Rate: _____ Attitude: _____

Femoral Pulse: _____ Character: _____

Mucous Membrane Color: _____ Capillary Refill Time (secs): _____ Hydration: _____

Color & Consistency of Feces on Thermometer: _____

Body Weight (lbs): _____ Body Condition: Normal / Overweight / Underweight

System Review

Integumentary	Otic	Ophthalmic	Musculoskeletal
__ Normal	__ Normal	__ Normal	__ Normal
__ Abnormal	__ Abnormal	__ Abnormal	__ Abnormal

Nervous	Cardiovascular	Respiratory	Digestive
__ Normal	__ Normal	__ Normal	__ Normal
__ Abnormal	__ Abnormal	__ Abnormal	__ Abnormal

Lymphatic	Reproductive	Urinary
__ Normal	__Normal	__Normal
__ Abnormal	__Abnormal	__Abnormal

Tests Performed:

_____CBC _____Clin Chem _____UA _____Fecal _____Micro

Describe Abnormal:

Signature:_____Date:_____

Figure 4.7 A clinical examination record is used to document health examinations. This may include arrival exams, study-related exams, exams for problems reported by staff, and annual physical exams for dogs kept long term.

to restrain the dog (Figure 4.8). A typical examination that assesses major organ systems and senses (integument, otic, ophthalmic, musculoskeletal, nervous, cardiovascular, respiratory, digestive, lymphatic, reproductive, and urinary) is as follows:

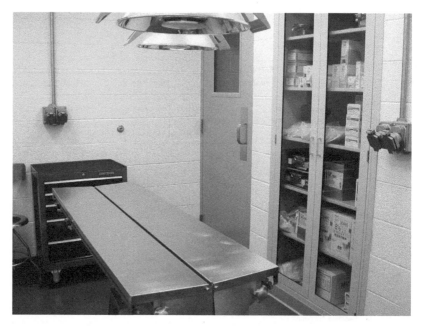

Figure 4.8 Examination room. A quiet examination room with overhead lights and an adjustable height examination table is preferred for evaluating dogs.

- Perform a general assessment of the animal's body condition and behavior (mental alertness, activity level, etc.) based on observations of the animal in its home cage, during the initial part of the examination (when the animal may be excited), as well as observations made during the course of the examination (when the animal may be calm). It is important to determine if the animal is calm, nervous, or fractious and restrain it accordingly.

- At the cage level, assess the animal's intake and output by observing food and water consumption (check bowls), the feces (quantity, characteristics, consistency, color, odor, etc.), and urine (quantity, characteristics, color, etc.).

- Obtain the animal's body weight and note the general body condition (under-, over-, or normal body weight).

- Verify the animal's identification by comparing the identification listed in the animal's arrival medical records with that on the animal (tattoo or identification tag). Note the breed and any identifying markings.

- Perform a basic vital signs check. This includes measuring body temperature, pulse/heart rate, and respiration rate (TPR). Normal body temperature for dogs is 101.5 ± 1°F and this may be increased by 1°F to 2°F during handling when dogs become excited. When measuring the body temperature, observe the feces on the thermometer and note the quantity and characteristics. Feces may be obtained at this time for parasite examinations and bacterial cultures.

- Measure the heart rate by auscultation of the thorax using a stethoscope and counting the heartbeats. Listen to both sides of the thorax; note the heart's rhythm, the intensity of the heart beats, and any abnormal sounds, such as a murmur. In order to detect pulse deficits, simultaneously count the femoral pulse (to compare with the heart rate) by placing one's index and middle fingers over the femoral artery. Measurement of the heart rate may be difficult when a dog becomes excited, in which case indicate "excited" on the exam form and recheck later. In these instances, checking the pulse when the dog is inside its cage provides resting heart rates.

- Measure the respiratory rate by auscultation of the thorax using a stethoscope and counting the number of respirations. Listen to both sides of the thorax, from top to bottom and front to back, noting the rate and rhythm of the inspirations and expirations as well as any abnormal sounds in an area, or absence thereof. Measurement of the respiratory rate may be difficult when a dog becomes excited, in which case indicate "panting" on the exam form and recheck later. In these instances, visual observation of the dog from outside its cage provides accurate resting respiratory rates.

- To further assess cardiovascular and pulmonary function, open the dog's mouth and observe the mucous membrane color (pink to red is normal). Also, assess the capillary refill time (CRT) by gently pressing a finger on the gums with enough pressure to blanche them and then count the amount of time needed for normal color to return to the gums (less than 1.5 seconds is normal).

- Examine the oral cavity for proper dentition, dental problems (e.g., tartar, calculus, gum disease, etc.), or other abnormalities.

- Examine the head and neck area by gentle palpation and direct visual observation. The skin should be examined for hair loss, lesions, and inflammation. Normal coats are soft and lustrous.

- Examine the eyes for redness, swelling, discharge, and opacities. Use a penlight to measure pupil size (equal size is normal) and pupillary light response (PLR) and perform additional testing (ophthalmoscope) as needed. A normal PLR is seen when the pupils of both eyes constrict when a light is shined in one eye. The response in the eye where the light is shined is a direct PLR and the response in the other eye is the indirect PLR. Test for direct and indirect PLRs in each eye.

- Examine the ears by direct observation for abnormal discharges or odors and masses. Use an otoscope to check the external ear canal and eardrum.

- Examine the nose for any discharges and normal flow of air (patency).

- Palpate the neck area for masses (enlarged lymph nodes or salivary glands) or musculoskeletal abnormalities.

- Hydration status can be partially assessed when measuring the CRT by noting the relative wetness or dryness of the gums, by tenting the skin of the neck and watching for it to return to normal position, and by observing the cornea, which should glisten normally.

- Superficially palpate the skin over the thorax and abdomen to check the skin for injuries, masses, or ectoparasites. Perform additional testing for ectoparasites as indicated (e.g., skin scrapes for mites).

- Palpate the legs and tail to check the skin for injuries, masses, or ectoparasites. Palpate superficial lymph nodes (e.g., axillary, inguinal, and popliteal) and the muscles and bones of the tail, legs, feet, and toes for abnormalities. Trim any overgrown nails.

- Deeply palpate (gently) the abdomen from front to back and top to bottom, assessing the internal organs for pain, masses, distension, or other abnormalities.

- Examine the penis for any discharges and the testicles for masses or cryptorchidism. Examine the perineum for urine or fecal staining and the vulva for discharges. Examine the rectum for discharges and perform a digital rectal exam to check the prostate or cervix/uterus. Examine the bitch's teats for swelling or discharge.

- Perform clinical laboratory tests. This commonly includes a complete blood count (CBC), clinical chemistry, urinalysis, and a fecal exam for parasites.

- Perform additional tests based on clinical signs of abnormalities or based on standard protocol. Additional testing may include an electrocardiogram (EKG), ultrasound, microbiological cultures and sensitivities, breeding soundness exams, etc.

Clinical Signs of Illness in Dogs

Clinical signs of illness in dogs are similar to those signs observed in many other species. It is important that the individuals observing the dogs (animal care staff, research investigators) be properly trained to observe animals in order to identify not only the general signs of illness but also the more subtle signs.

- Decreased appetite or thirst as noted by decreased feed or water consumption.
- Change in activity level, such as reflex withdrawal, biting at a source of pain or an affected area, increased activity, aversive behavior toward cage mates, or decreased activity.
- Change in posture, such as recumbent, hunched with head tucked into abdomen, standing with front legs apart, or "sleeping" posture.
- Change in temperament, such as more or less docile or aggressive, quiet, unsociable, or depressed and unresponsive.
- Restlessness, such as shaking or scratching a particular area, hyperactive, or circling.
- Vocalization, such as squealing, moaning, or barking when alone or during handling when pressure is exerted on the affected area.
- Change in appearance, such as weight loss, sunken abdomen, or dehydration.
- Changes in the eyes, such as sunken with or without discharge, almost closed, or exudates.
- Changes in locomotion, such as stilted gait, lameness, or immobility.
- Changes in urination, such as increased or decreased urination or incontinence.
- Changes in respiration, such as increased respiratory rate, labored breathing, "chattering," or nasal discharge.
- General changes such as hypothermia (cool to the touch), hyperthermia (fever), or weight loss.

common clinical problems

Reviewed in this section are common clinical problems one might encounter in dogs used in research settings. Importantly, many of the classic dog diseases (e.g., viral or endoparasites) are much less common in modern lab settings due to improved management practices regarding sourcing choices (e.g., obtaining purpose-bred dogs from reputable vendors with comprehensive veterinary care programs versus random-source dogs), housing methods (indoor versus outdoor), institutional health care, sanitation, and staff training programs. It is also critical to distinguish between primary clinical problems and those related to the ongoing research, as treatment options may differ significantly. In these instances, it is important to consult with a veterinarian and the research investigator, as clinical signs associated with the research being performed may not be treatable.

Trained staff are better able to report sick animals sooner and identify subtle clinical signs, including those that may be study-related effects of great consequence. For additional information on potential clinical problems, it is recommended that the standard references be consulted, including *The Merck Veterinary Manual* series (Merck & Co., Whitehouse Station, NJ), *Clinical Microbiology and Infectious Diseases of the Dog and Cat* (W.B. Saunders, Philadelphia), *Infectious Diseases of the Dog and Cat* (W.B. Saunders, Philadelphia), and *Laboratory Animal Medicine*, 2nd edition (Academic Press, San Diego).[1-4]

Viral Diseases

Canine parvovirus

In susceptible populations, canine parvovirus (CPV) generally presents clinically as a form of gastroenteritis. As the virus has a predilection for rapidly dividing cells, notably those of the intestine, bone marrow, and lymphoid tissues, clinical signs of disease are attributable to direct damage or death to these cells and the sequelae thereof. These include vomiting, diarrhea (often hemorrhagic), loss of appetite, fluid and electrolyte loss, lethargy, fever, and leukopenia. While all ages may be infected, neonates are most susceptible to disease due to the waning of protective maternal antibodies prior to protection from vaccination. Transmission occurs by direct (fecal-oral route) and indirect (fomites) contact, and shedding of the virus can last for up to 3 weeks after infection. Recovered dogs serve as carriers. Diagnosis is by clinical signs and by commercial enzyme-linked immunosorbent assay (ELISA) tests of fecal samples. Treatment is primarily supportive (fluids and electrolytes) and most dogs recover in a few days. Vaccination is key to the prevention and control of parvovirus (Figure 4.9). As parvovirus is able to survive for long periods of time in the environment and is resistant to temperature extremes and many common disinfectants, it is important to use disinfectants with known efficacy against the virus (e.g., bleach) during decontamination efforts. Dogs should be quarantined during treatment.

Canine distemper

Disease due to canine distemper virus (CDV) varies in severity based on the virulence of the strain of virus. Milder forms are characterized by respiratory signs, while more severe forms of the disease have systemic effects, notably to the lungs, gastrointestinal tract, skin, and CNS, often accompanied by secondary bacterial infections. Clinical signs include coughing, oculonasal discharge, diarrhea, vomiting, fever, and hyperkeratosis of the footpad (hard pad disease). Neurological problems range from muscle twitching to ataxia, ascending paresis, paralysis, and convulsions. Transmission is by aerosol drop-

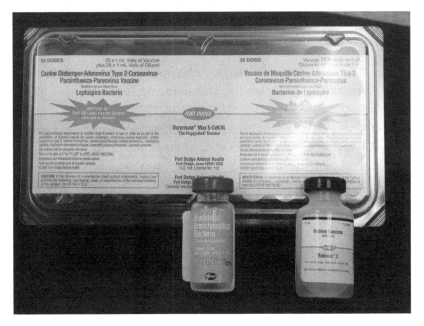

Figure 4.9 Canine vaccines. Maintaining vaccinations begun at the vendor is recommended as good preventive medicine, reducing the incidence of common viral diseases in dogs.

lets and shedding can continue for months after infection. Diagnosis is by clinical signs (fever with multisystemic signs including neurological signs). Important differential diagnoses include kennel cough and rabies. Treatment involves supportive modalities, including fluids, electrolytes, and antibiotics. Vaccination is key to the prevention and control of distemper virus. Canine distemper virus is unstable in the environment and susceptible to many disinfectants. Dogs should be quarantined during treatment, however, humane euthanasia may be preferred in research settings.

Canine coronavirus

Disease due to canine coronavirus (CCV) generally manifests itself as a mild gastroenteritis that may include a yellow-brown diarrhea. Infections may be subclinical and the disease is usually self-limiting. Definitive diagnosis is often unnecessary. Transmission is by direct contact (fecal-oral route). Vaccination is the key to prevention and control of CCV infections.

Rabies

All mammals are susceptible to the rhabdovirus that causes rabies, and infection by the causative virus leads to a rapidly fatal encephalitis. Stages of the disease include:

- The prodromal stage, characterized by behavioral changes including irritability, anorexia, aggressiveness, altered vocalizations, and preference for solitude;
- The excitative or furious stage, where animals become very alert, irrational, and aggressive, often seeking out victims; and
- The paralytic stage, where the throat and mouth become paralyzed, and profuse drooling, an inability to swallow, and a dropped jaw may be observed.

Death usually occurs within 10 days of the onset of clinical signs. Transmission is primarily by direct contact (saliva, bite). Diagnosis is made by clinical signs and immunofluorescence of virus in brain tissues. Important differentials include other CNS disorders such as distemper, bacterial encephalitis, and underlying hepatic disease. Vaccination and limiting exposure to potential carriers are keys to the prevention and control of rabies in animals. Workers at risk should consider preexposure immunization. In a research setting, humane euthanasia of suspected animals is often preferred rather than isolation and waiting for the development of signs. Rabies is rare in purpose-bred dogs but should always be considered in random-source dogs. A purpose-bred dog is normally isolated and monitored following a human bite incident, and a random-source dog is usually euthanized and tested.

Kennel cough

Infectious tracheobronchitis (kennel cough) is a contagious, but generally self-limiting disease of the respiratory tract in dogs. More severe forms of the disease include chronic bronchitis and bronchopneumonia. Potential etiologic agents, alone or in combination, include canine parainfluenza virus (PAV), canine adenovirus 1 and 2 (CAV 1 and 2), canine distemper virus, *Bordetella bronchiseptica*, canine herpes virus, canine reoviruses 1, 2, and 3, and *Mycoplasma* sp. Concurrent infections by multiple agents and secondary bacterial infections following viral infection are common. In the self-limiting, milder form of the disease, a dry, hacking cough that may progress to a purulent nasal discharge and gagging/retching is observed. Fever, depression, and anorexia are observed during more severe forms of the disease, which suggests multiple agent involvement and has a poorer prognosis, including death. Diagnosis is usually based on clinical signs. Supportive treatment and isolation are generally adequate for milder forms of kennel cough, but cough suppressants and antibiotics (especially when bacterial causes are identified) may be indicated. Vaccination is a key to prevention and proper isolation of sick animals and sanitation of contaminated areas is important in controlling the spread of the disease.

Bacterial Diseases

Leptospirosis

Leptospirosis is a contagious disease of animals and man of all ages that varies in severity from subclinical infections to severe disease. The causative agents are multiple serovars of the spirochete *Leptospira interrogans sensu lato*, including *pomona*, *grippotyphosa*, *canicola*, and *icterohemorraghiae*. Clinical signs may be nonspecific and include depression, fever, and pain or may be related to target organ damage (kidneys and liver), such as uremia, dehydration, hemoglobinuria, vomiting, diarrhea, oral ulcers, and bleeding disorders. Transmission is from breaks in the skin, mucosal penetration, or ingestion of contaminated water. Recovered animals may be carriers and can shed for months to years. Diagnosis is based on clinical signs and finding spirochetes in urine samples. Treatment is as for renal or liver disease and includes supportive fluids, electrolytes, and antibiotics. Vaccination is available for some serovars of leptospira, but these are not cross protective against infection by other serovars. Control efforts should be directed toward limiting exposure to carriers or sources of contamination.

Parasitic Diseases

Protozoa

Dogs may be infected by a variety of gastrointestinal protozoa. Giardiasis results from infection by *Giardia duodenalis* (*lamblia*). Inapparent infections are most common, however, diarrhea may occur with heavier infections. Transmission is direct by consumption of contaminated food or water and the diagnosis is based on clinical signs and observation of giardia cysts in fecal samples. Metronidazole (25 to 30 mg/kg orally once a day for 5 to 10 days) and supportive fluids are commonly used to treat giardiasis. Prevention and control measures include good sanitation practices and disinfection of contaminated areas with bleach or a quaternary ammonium compound.

Coccidiosis in dogs is associated with infection by *Cystoisospora canis*, *Cystoisospora ohioensis*, *Cystoisospora burrowsi*, or *Cystoisospora neorivolta*. Clinical signs, transmission, diagnosis, prevention, and control measures are similar to those for giardia. As infections are usually self-limiting, treatment may not be necessary. Treatment options include sulfadimethoxine (25 to 30 mg/lb. orally once a day for 10 days) and trimethoprim sulfa (15 mg/lb. orally once a day for 10 days).

Nematodes

Research dogs are susceptible to infection by a variety of nematodes. However, acquisition of only purpose-bred dogs minimizes the risk of acquiring these parasites. Nematodes causing intestinal disease include hookworms (*Ancylostoma caninum*), ascarids (*Toxacara canis*), whipworms (*Trichuris vulpis*), and strongyloides (*Strongyloides stercoralis*). Clinical signs range from none to diarrhea, vomiting, dehydration, lethargy, loss of appetite, and weight loss. Hookworm infections can produce a bloody diarrhea and anemia from blood loss. Diagnosis is by detecting worms or parasite eggs in the feces. Prevention and control measures include limiting exposure to infected animals, good sanitation to eliminate eggs or larvae, and prophylactic treatment with anthelmintics.

Most dogs with heartworm infections (*Dirofilaria immitis*) show no clinical signs. Severely and chronically infected dogs may exhibit coughing, dyspnea, exercise intolerance, and heart failure. Diagnosis is by detection of adult heartworm antigen or microfilaria (immature heartworms) from blood samples. Prevention and control measures include limiting exposure to mosquitoes and placing dogs on prophylactic treatment with anthelmintics, especially when outdoor housing is used. Treatment of dogs infected with heartworms may be prohibitive in research settings and acquisition of heartworm-free animals is preferred.

Cestodes

Tapeworm infections in research dogs can be minimized or excluded by acquiring only purpose-bred dogs and subsequently limiting access to intermediate host vectors through indoor housing. Tapeworms of primary concern include *Diplydium caninum*, *Taenia pisiformis*, and less commonly, *Echinococcus granulosus*. Clinical signs are uncommon, but may include diarrhea, loss of appetite, and weight loss. Diagnosis is made by detection of eggs or tapeworm segments (proglottids) in the feces. Prevention and control includes limiting access to vectors (fleas and lice for *Diplydium*, rodents and rabbits for *Taenia*, etc.) and treatment of active flea/lice infections. Dogs already infected with tapeworms may be effectively treated with praziquantel.

Arthropods

Fleas

Dogs are most commonly infested by *Ctenocephalides felis*, the cat flea (see Figure 2.3). Dogs may also become infested with *Ctenocephalides canis*, the dog flea, *Pulex irritans*, and *Echidnophaga gallinacea*. Fleas can infest man and fleas may act as vectors for other pathogens (including tapeworms and hemoprotozoa). Clinical signs range from localized alopecia and pruritus (hot spots) in acute infections, to widespread papules, crusting, and hyperpigmentation over the tail, head, lower back, and thighs. Pruritus with licking and biting of the skin is common to flea allergy dermatitis (FAD), a hypersensitivity reaction to proteins in flea saliva. Diagnosis is by clinical signs and observation of flea dirt (feces) or fleas on the animal. Prevention through acquisition of purpose-bred dogs is important in research settings. Control involves thorough and concurrent environmental cleanup of eggs and treatment of dogs using topical insecticides and juvenile growth regulators. Steroids or antibiotics are used to treat hot spots and FAD.

Mites

Dogs infected with *Demodex canis* may develop demodicosis. Because demodex mites are commonly transmitted to pups during nursing, demodex mites are considered normal fauna for dogs and are not contagious to man. Localized demodicosis is characterized by focal alopecia that generally resolves spontaneously. Generalized demodicosis can be severe, with widespread alopecia, papules, pustules, hyperpigmentation, and crusting of the skin. Diagnosis is based on clinical signs and from observation of mites in skin scrapings. Treatment and control includes the use of oral ivermectin or milbemycin, and for more severe generalized disease, amitraz dips. Stress and other systemic disease exacerbates demodicosis. Dogs with generalized demodicosis should not be used for research and should be removed from the colony.

Dogs infected with *Sarcoptes scabiei* var. *canis* develop sarcoptic mange (scabies). Because sarcoptic mange mites live on and off the host, they are contagious to man and other dogs. Clinical signs include acute onset of severe pruritus, with papules (early) and excoriations with thick crusting of the skin over affected areas, most commonly the ventral abdomen, chest, ears, and legs. Diagnosis is based on clinical signs and from observation of mites in deep skin scrapings. Treatment and control includes oral ivermectin or milbemycin.

Lice

Dogs may be infected by the sucking louse *Linognathus setosus* and by the biting lice *Trichodectes canis* and *Heterodoxus spiniger*. Pediculosis may be asymptomatic or result in pruritus, alopecia, papules, crusting, and excoriation of the skin. Transmission is by direct contact. Because lice are host specific, they are not infectious to man. Diagnosis is by clinical signs or the observation of lice eggs (nits) on hair shafts or lice on the dog. Prevention and control measures include the use of only purpose-bred dogs. Treatment options include insecticidal shampoos and dips.

Ticks

Dogs may be infected by various species of *Rhipecephalus*, *Ixodes*, and *Dermacentor* ticks. Examples include *Rhipecephalus sanguineus* (brown dog tick), *Dermacenter variabilis* (American dog tick), and *Amblyomma maculatum* (Gulf Coast tick). By themselves, ticks are generally inapparent, although neurotoxins contained in tick saliva can result in an ascending, flaccid paralysis. However, ticks serve as vectors for many infectious pathogens such as *Rickettsia rickettsi*a (the causative agent of Rocky Mountain spotted fever), *Borrellia burgdorferi* (the causative agent of Lyme disease), *Ehrlichia canis* (ehrlichiosis), *Babesia canis* (babesiosis), *Hemobartonella canis* (hemobartonellosis), and *Hepatazoon canis* (hepatozoonosis). Prevention and control measures include the use of purpose-bred dogs and the use of indoor housing facilities. Removal of the entire tick is important and can reverse the early stages of tick-induced paralysis. Outdoor housed dogs may be treated with prophylactic topical insecticides.

Fungal Diseases

Dogs are susceptible to various fungi that may result in localized or systemic disease. The use of purpose-bred dogs should prevent most fungal disease. Ringworm, or dermatophytosis, is caused by *Microsporum canis*, *Microsporum gypseum*, or *Trichophyton mentagrophytes*. Ringworm lesions are typically outward spreading, circular, raised, red lesions with a central area of alopecia. Because dermatophytes are ubiquitous in the environment and very contagious, they can be readily spread between dogs and man. Topical treatments are generally used. Other fungal diseases due to *Blastomyces dermatidis*, *Histoplasma capsulatum*, *Coccidiodes immitis*, or *Cryptococcus neoformans* var. *neoformans* are less common in laboratory settings.

Miscellaneous Diseases and Conditions

Interdigital cysts

Interdigital cysts may be seen in research colony dogs. Clinical signs include reddened, swollen areas between the toes with an initial observation of lameness in the affected leg or licking of the affected foot. The cause is unknown, but chronic interdigital dermatitis, age, body condition score, and type of flooring have been described recently as possible causes.[5] Treatment options include cleaning the area with a disinfectant, foot soaks in warm water with an antiseptic solution, topical or oral antibiotics, and anti-inflammatory agents.

Recurrent cysts or those refractory to treatment may require surgical removal. Kovacs et al.[5] recommend consideration of the type of flooring used for dogs during renovation or new construction. Personal experience with a raised slatted floor system suggests they are beneficial as a preventative measure.[1,5]

Juvenile polyarteritis syndrome: beagle pain syndrome

This condition has been reported in research colony dogs, primarily beagles. Clinical signs include a progression from pain when opening the mouth, grunting when being lifted, and a standing posture characterized by an arched back, extended neck, lowered head, and stiff gait. Oral mucosa may be reddened, appetite is often depressed, and body temperature may be elevated to between 104°F and 106°F. Neutrophilia and necrotizing arteritis are characteristic findings. Chronic cases may result in muscular atrophy of the head and neck and weight loss. More often, the signs occur intermittently and recurrence is common. Signs are initially observed when handling the dog and the cause is unknown. Treatment with antibiotics and anti-inflammatory drugs may provide temporary control, but recurrence upon withdrawal of medications is reported.[6–8]

Cherry eye

Protrusion of the gland of the nictitating membrane (the third eyelid) is commonly referred to as "cherry eye" (Figure 4.10). Clinically, a red mass is observed in the medial (nasal) aspect of the eye. Prolonged exposure of this tissue may result in drying or damage to the gland or damage to the cornea. The cause of cherry eye is unknown and

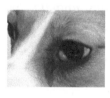

if not self-resolving, treatment options range from topical or systemic antibiotics or corticosteroids to surgical reduction or removal. Because this gland provides lubrication to the eye through production of tears, one should assess this potential risk prior to removal of the gland.[1,9,10]

Figure 4.10 Cherry eye.

Dental conditions

Various dental conditions may occur in research colony dogs, some of which may affect ongoing research in addition to the animal's health. Examples include malocclusion, retained deciduous teeth, plaque, calculus, periodontal disease, tooth root abscess, and fractured teeth. Contributing factors include inadequate dental care programs, genetics, and diet (soft versus hard food, high fat content, etc.). Treatment should be based on the clinical condition. Implementation of a prophylactic dental care program such as manual or ultrasonic scaling as part of the facility's overall canine preventive medicine program is recommended and invaluable, especially for dogs maintained long term.[11,12]

Obesity

Obesity in research dogs is not uncommon, yet it is often overlooked. Because obesity is associated with multiple health problems (cardiovascular disease, musculoskeletal problems, diabetes, etc.), research implications may be profound. Caging requirements, limited exercise, genetics, *ad libitum* versus measured feedings or feedings that meet energy requirements, hypothyroidism, spay/neuter, and maintaining dog colonies for longer periods of time are some potential causative factors. Generally people and animals are considered to be obese when they are 20% to 25% over the ideal weight for their body type. Subjectively, a dog of normal weight should have ribs that are barely discernable yet easily palpated. Treatments should be directed at potential underlying causes (e.g., thyroid deficiency). Otherwise, weight reduction programs should be implemented, including restricted diets, increased activity, or a change in diet. Diet restrictions reducing calories and energy content should be gradual to produce a steady and sustainable weight loss. Subsequently, body weight assessments should be performed at regular intervals.[13]

Implant problems

Dogs are used in a variety of research projects that utilize implants. Telemetry implants, vascular access ports, indwelling vascular or biliary cannula, and intestinal access ports are some examples. Microchip implants for identification purposes may also be a source of implant problems. Because properly placed and maintained implants may last for many months, it is imperative to follow strict aseptic procedures during implantation, maintenance of the implant and the implantation site, and experimental use of the implant. Otherwise, the most likely outcome will be removal of the implant due to infection or improper function. Localized skin infections may be treated using topical antibiotics and wound cleaning, however, systemic antibiotics, based on empirical data or culture and sensitivity testing of blood, may be needed when more aggressive treatment is required or if septicemia is a potential concern. Ultimately, prompt removal of the implant supplemented with an extended regimen of systemic antibiotics is the only definitive treatment option.

Traumatic injuries

Traumatic injuries from various causes such as aggressive play, caging defects, and implants that cause local irritation or abscess formation may occur. Prompt attention through regular reporting of injuries by staff to the veterinarian will minimize the impact and lead to quicker, less complicated resolution of the problem. Basic wound care procedures should be followed. Uncomplicated wound care includes clipping the fur in the surrounding area, cleaning the area with antiseptics (povidone-iodine or chlorhexidine solution), application of topical antibiotics, and bandaging the wound. More complicated wounds may require local or general anesthesia, surgical debridement, and wound closure, although contaminated, draining wounds are better left open or should have delayed closure. Systemic antibiotics, selected based on empirical data or culture and sensitivity testing of the wound, are standard procedure for deeper wounds. Dogs with wounds should receive regular evaluation and bandage changes.

Behavioral disorders

Dogs with abnormal or aberrant behaviors may be encountered in research settings. These behaviors may result from inadequate socialization when young, from stress related to research use, from specific test compounds, or from genetic predisposition. Because dogs with behavioral disorders may pose safety risks to people, other dogs, or themselves, they may be unsuitable for research. It is important to identify vendors that have robust enrichment programs, since such programs result in well-socialized research animals.

treatment of diseases

Treatment of disease should be performed under the direction of a veterinarian. Consideration of research implications should be part of treatment decisions, as should consultation with research staff. Diagnostic testing should be performed, but often symptomatic treatment must be initiated prior to making a clear diagnosis. Treatment of some general conditions is described below. Tables 4.1 through 4.4

list common antibiotic, antifungal, antiparasitic, and miscellaneous drugs used to treat dogs.

General Treatment of Diarrhea

Diarrhea can occur from multiple causes, including viral or bacterial pathogens, intestinal parasites, pancreatic, intestinal, or hepatic disease, dietary problems, or study-related causes. Often the presentation is nonspecific, at least initially, or the causative factor remains undiagnosed while the animal remains symptomatic. While one should pursue a diagnosis, in the absence of a clear diagnosis, one should begin treating the animal based on the symptoms. Standard

TABLE 4.1: COMMON ANTIBIOTIC DRUGS FOR THE DOG

Antibiotic drug	Suggested dose	References
Amoxicillin	10 mg/kg PO BID	16
Cephalexin	35 mg/kg PO every 12 hours	16
Cephalothin	40–80 mg/kg day IM, IV every 8–12 hours	16
Clavamox	14 mg/kg PO BID	16
Enrofloxacin	2.5–5 mg/kg PO BID	16
Gentamicin	2–4 mg/kg SC, IM every 12 hours the first day, then SID	16
Trimethoprim (TMP)/sulfadiazine	15 mg/kg PO BID	16
Tetracycline	10–25 mg/kg PO BID or TID	16

BID, twice a day; IM, intramuscular; IV, intravenous; PO (per os), oral dose; SC, subcutaneous; SID, once a day; TID, three times a day.

TABLE 4.2: COMMON ANTIFUNGAL DRUGS FOR THE DOG

Antifungal drug	Suggested dose	References
Amphotericin B	0.25–0.5 mg/kg two to three times a week slow IV drip with dextrose and saline	16
Fluconazole	2.5 mg/kg BID	2
Griseofulvin	20 mg/kg PO SID	16
Ketoconazole	10–20 mg/kg PO every 8–12 hours	16

BID, twice a day; IV, intravenous; PO (per os), oral dose; SID, once a day.

TABLE 4.3: COMMON ANTIPARASITIC DRUGS FOR THE DOG

Antiparasitic drug	Suggested dose	Indication	References
Fenbendazole	50 mg/kg PO SID for 3 days	Helminths	16
Ivermectin	6 µg/kg PO monthly	Heartworm prevention	16
Mebendazole	22 mg/kg PO SID for 3 days	Helminths	16
Metronidazole	60 mg/kg PO SID for 5 days	Giardiasis	16
Praziquantel	1/2 tablet per 2.5 kg PO, maximum 5 tablets	Tapeworms	16
Pyrantel pamoate	5 mg/kg PO, repeat in 7 days	Helminths	16

PO (per os), oral dose; SC, subcutaneous; SID, once a day.

TABLE 4.4: MISCELLANEOUS DRUGS FOR THE DOG

Therapeutic agent	Suggested dose	References
Dexamethasone	1–5 mg/kg slow IV infusion	16
Prednisolone	0.5–2.0 mg/kg PO	16
Prednisone	0.5–2.0 mg/kg PO	16

IV, intravenous; PO (per os), oral dose.

practices include withholding food for 24 hours, after which time the animal can be returned to its regular diet or to a bland diet (rice) in reduced quantities. Fluid deficits should be monitored. If the animal can maintain hydration through oral fluid intake, supplementation may not be needed. If vomiting prevents oral intake or if diarrhea is too profuse, fluids can be administered subcutaneously or intravenously. Kaopectate (Pfizer Consumer Healthcare, New York, NY) can be used as an absorbant/protectant, and antimotility drugs such as Lomotil (G.D. Searle LLC, Chicago, IL) may be considered for more severe cases.[14,15]

General Treatment of Dehydration

Dogs can become dehydrated from study-related effects, water supply problems, or various constitutive disease conditions such as diarrhea. Pending diagnostic test results, it is important to initiate replacement therapy before fluid deficits become severe. Dehydration can be assessed by assessing the dryness of the cornea or the tackiness of the oral mucosal, or by the skin tent test, whereby skin in the dorsal neck area is pulled up and released. Normally, tented skin will return within 1 second of release; longer return times equate to increased levels of dehydration. Common fluids used as replacement therapy include 0.9% saline and lactated Ringers solution. Routes of administration may be oral, subcutaneous, or intravenous, depending on the ease of administration, ability to retain the fluids, fractiousness of the animal, or extent of dehydration.[14]

General Treatment of Anorexia

Dogs may experience anorexia for various reasons and frequently the cause is unknown or is study related. Returning the animal back to consumption of a normal amount of food may be difficult, but it is important to do so promptly for the animal's general health and study-related reasons. Strategies to return the animal to feed include enticing the animal to eat a preferred, highly palatable food, such as canned dog food. Similarly, dog biscuits or peanut butter are considered desirable by many dogs. Nutri-Cal (EVSCO, Libertyville, IL) is a calorie-dense nutritional supplement that can be placed in the animal's mouth or on the face which is then consumed during subsequent grooming activity by the animal. During periods of anorexia, it is important to regularly weigh the animal and ensure that normal water intake is maintained.[14]

Drug Dosages in Dogs

Medications should be provided under the direction of a veterinarian following diagnostic evaluation. Tables 4.1 through 4.4 list dosing regimens for drugs commonly used for dogs, but the age, sex, nutritional and physical status, and history of experimental use of the animal may affect results.

disease prevention through sanitation

Proper sanitation practices and procedures are fundamental activities critical for disease prevention and control. Dog kennels and cages, feeders, water bowls, and enrichment devices should be cleaned, disinfected, and sanitized regularly, as described in Chapter 2. Colony rooms should be regularly emptied and sanitized, along with all removable and fixed equipment. Feces, urine, soiled food, and soiled bedding materials should be removed daily. Instruments and equipment used to clean cages or manipulate animals should be properly cleaned and disinfected after use. Personnel caring for or working with dogs should wear appropriate clothing and personal protective equipment (PPE), such as scrubs and disposable garments (lab coats, gloves, masks, etc.), over scrubs or street clothes. All personnel should follow standard hygienic practices, including washing hands with disinfectant soap after handling animals and before leaving the animal room.[17]

anesthesia, analgesia, and sedation

Anesthesia, analgesia, and sedation/tranquilization are routinely performed in research settings. The purpose of this section is to describe basic procedures involved in performing canine anesthesia from the preoperative period through postoperative recovery. Information on selected anesthetics, analgesics, sedatives/tranquilizers, and other emergency drugs used in dogs are listed in Tables 4.5 through 4.8. One should account for individual animal variation when using anesthetics based on age, sex, strain, physical status, and history of experimental use. It is recommended that one uses a dose at the lower end of the recommended range until they becomes familiar with

TABLE 4.5: COMMON PREANESTHETIC AND ANESTHETIC DRUGS FOR THE DOG

Therapeutic agent	Suggested dose	Indication	References
Acepromazine	0.1–0.5 mg/kg IV, IM to 3 mg maximum	Tranquilizer	20, 21
Atipamezole	50–400 µg/kg IM, IV	Reversal agent	20, 21
Atropine	0.05 mg/kg IM, SC	Anticholinergic	16, 20, 21
Buprenorphine	0.01–0.02 mg/kg SC	Analgesic	20, 21, 23, 24
Diazepam	1–2 mg/kg IV to 20 mg maximum	Tranquilizer	16
Glycopyrrolate	0.01–0.02 mg/kg SC, IM	Anticholinergic	20, 21, 23, 24
Medetomidine	0.1–0.8 mg/kg IM, SC, IV	Tranquilizer	20, 21
Midazolam	0.7–0.22 mg/kg IM, IV	Tranquilizer	16

IM, intramuscular; IV, intravenous; SC, subcutaneous.

TABLE 4.6: COMMON INJECTABLE ANESTHETIC DRUGS FOR THE DOG

Therapeutic agent	Suggested dose	References
Pentobarbital	20–30 mg/kg IV	19–21
Propofol	5–7.5 mg/kg IV induction, then 0.2–0.4 mg/kg/min constant rate infusion or 1–2 mg/kg IV incremental maintenance doses	19–21
Thiopental	10–20 mg/kg IV	19–21

IV, intravenous.

TABLE 4.7: COMMON ANALGESIC DRUGS FOR THE DOG

Analgesic agent	Suggested dose	References
Aspirin	10–20 mg/kg PO every 12 hours	16, 23, 24
Bupivicaine	Local infiltration of area	16
Buprenorphine	0.01–0.02 mg/kg SC every 12 hours	16, 20, 21, 23, 24
Butorphanol	0.2–0.4 mg/kg SC, IM, IV every 2–5 hours	16, 20, 21, 23, 24
Carprofen	1–2 mg/kg PO BID	20, 21, 24
Fentanyl	0.04–0.08 mg/kg SC, IM, IV every 1–2 hours	20, 21, 24
Fentanyl patch	25, 50, 75, and 100 μg sizes	24
Ketoprofen	2 mg/kg IM	24
Lidocaine 1%	Local infiltration of area	20, 21
Morphine	0.1 mg/kg SC every 4 hours	16
Oxymorphone	0.2 mg/kg SC, IV	16

BID, twice a day; IM, intramuscular; IV, intravenous; PO (per os), oral dose; SC, subcutaneous.

TABLE 4.8: COMMON EMERGENCY DRUGS FOR THE DOG

Therapeutic agent	Suggested dose	Indication	References
Aminophylline	10 mg/kg IM, IV	Bronchodilator	16, 23, 24
Dipyrone	28 mg/kg IM, SC, IV TID	Antipyretic, analgesic	28
Dopamine	2–15 μg/kg/min IV	Positive ionotrope	16
Doxapram	5–10 mg/kg IV, repeat in 15–20 minutes	Respiratory stimulant	23, 24
Epinephrine 1:10,000	0.5–1.5 ml IV every 30 minutes	Positive ionotrope	16
Furosemide	2–4 mg/kg PO every 12 hours	Diuretic	16
Naloxone	0.2–0.4 mg IM, SC, IV	Opioid reversal	16

IM, intramuscular; IV, intravenous; PO (per os), oral dose; SC, subcutaneous; TID, three times a day.

an anesthetic regimen. Consulting with a veterinarian and the use of available texts such as *Handbook of Veterinary Anesthesia* (C.V. Mosby, St. Louis), *Textbook of Small Animal Surgery*, 2nd edition (W.B. Saunders, Philadelphia), *Laboratory Animal Anesthesia*, 1st and 2nd editions (Academic Press, San Diego) on the subject to develop anesthesia regimens is strongly recommended.[18–22]

Common Definitions

- Analgesia is the loss of sensibility to pain.
- Anesthesia is the complete loss of feeling or sensation to a part of the body or the entire body. It is generally induced by a drug that results in depression of activity of nervous tissue locally, regionally, or to the entire body.
- Balanced anesthesia is surgical anesthesia accomplished through the use of two or more agents or anesthetic techniques that individually contribute their own pharmacologic effects.
- General anesthesia is anesthesia that results in the loss of consciousness and loss of sensation to the entire body. It includes muscle relaxation, analgesia, and decreased reflexes.
- Local anesthesia is anesthesia of a localized area.
- Sedation is a state of calmness and awakeness with mild CNS depression. Patients can be aroused with appropriate stimuli.
- Surgical anesthesia is the loss of consciousness and sensation with adequate analgesia and muscle relaxation such that the surgical procedure can be performed without movement or pain to the patient.
- Tranquilization is a state of tranquility and calmness where the patient is awake, relaxed, and calm. Analgesia is not usually present and patients can be aroused by use of appropriate stimuli.

principles of general anesthesia

General principles of anesthesia, as for other species, also apply to dogs. Proper patient selection, acclimation and preparation, use of facilities designed for canine surgery, adherence to principles of aseptic technique, good surgical and tissue handling techniques, comprehensive case management during the entire perioperative period, the level of experience and training of personnel performing anesthesia or surgery, and the use of analgesics are key elements to consider. Listed below are some basic considerations that should be followed when anesthetizing dogs.[18-22]

- Examine the dog in advance of the day of the procedure to assess its health status. This should include a physical to assess all major systems as well as supplemental tests such as a CBC, clinical chemistry, urinalysis, radiographs, etc. Problems suggestive of disease conditions may result in postponement of elective anesthesia procedures.

- Fasting of dogs for 8 to 12 hours prior to anesthesia is recommended, except for emergency procedures when time does not permit this. Fasting empties the stomach and helps prevent vomiting and aspiration during or after surgery. Ensuring that the dog has defecated and urinated prior to anesthesia is also recommended.

- Water generally can be offered up to the time when premedication for anesthesia is started. It is important to ensure the dog is properly hydrated and the risk of vomiting from drinking too much water prior to surgery is low. Certain procedures, such as gastric or intestinal surgery, may require earlier withdrawal of water.

- Shortly before the procedure, move the dog to a quiet area. Perform another brief examination to identify any changes from the prior comprehensive examination. Note the results of this examination on the anesthesia record, which should be started at this time.

- Obtain an accurate body weight. This is important for calculating the dosages of all drugs and fluids used, as well as for monitoring return to normal body weight following the procedure.

- Administer the calculated doses of preanesthetic medications (atropine, antibiotics, analgesics, etc.) about 30 to 60 minutes prior to induction of anesthesia. Tranquilizers or sedatives to help reduce anxiety and fear can be administered at this time.

- Obtain the animal's body temperature. It is important to monitor the animal's temperature in order to prevent hypothermia and to facilitate recovery. Excited dogs may have temperatures that are elevated 1°F to 2°F due to struggling, and this should be noted.

- Induce anesthesia and continue to monitor the depth of anesthesia regularly. This is done by checking and recording vital signs (temperature, pulse, respiration, pain perception) on the anesthesia/surgery record (Figure 4.11).

- Provide supplemental heat to the dog by placing a circulating warm-water heating pad under it, by covering it with a blanket, or a combination of the two. The ability to regulate body temperature is lost during general anesthesia, and without the provision of supplemental heat, delayed recovery or death may occur. This is more of a problem in smaller dogs, which have a higher surface area: body mass ratio and for longer procedures (longer than 15 to 20 minutes). Remove blankets when ready to scrub and drape for surgery.

Anesthesia / Surgery Record

This record must be completed by the investigator for inclusion in the individual animal's health record. The information requested below is necessary to ensure proper anesthetic monitoring.

Protocol Number_____Principal Investigator_____Extension_____

Investigator/Surgeon_____Assistant(s)_____Date of Procedure_____

Description of Procedure_____

PRE-OPERATIVE EVALUATION

Animal Information: Species_____Animal ID_____Animal Fasting (Y/N)_____

Body Weight_____Temperature_____Heart Rate_____Respiratory Rate_____

ANESTHETICS INFORMATION   (List All Agent(s), Doses (mg/kg), and Routes of Administration.)

Pre-Anesthetic(s)_____Induction_____

_____Induction Time_____

Maintenance_____

Fluids (Type, Route, Rate)_____Antibiotics_____

Time (minutes)		0	30	60	30	60	30	60	30	60	30	60	30
A	Anesthesia Start												
AA	Anesthesia End												
O	Procedure Start												
OO	Procedure End												
	300												
	280												
	260												
SYMBOLS	240												
H = Heart Rate	220												
	200												
R = Respiratory Rate	180												
	160												
	140												
	120												
	100												
	80												
	60												
	40												
	20												
Temperature													

Post Anesthetic / Post Operative Observations

Procedure/Surgery End Time_____Extubation Time_____Total Fluids_____(mls)

Analgesics: (List All Agent(s), Doses (mg/kg), Routes and Duration of Administration.)

Remarks: (Pre-Anesthesia/Pre-Op, Induction, Maintenance, Emergence, Post-Op, Recovery, and Complications.)

Figure 4.11 Anesthesia/surgery record form.

- Administer supplemental fluids and electrolytes to the dog, especially for procedures longer than 1 hour or when blood loss is expected or occurs. Fluid rates of 5 to 10 ml/lb/hour intravenously are normal, starting at initial induction through sternal recumbency postoperatively.

- Postanesthesia, maintain supplemental heat and continue to monitor the animal's vital signs regularly to ensure a full recovery. The frequency of monitoring can be reduced as the animal awakens and the heat source can be removed when it is fully awake.

- Begin administering postoperative analgesics. Assessment of clinical signs and recovery from the procedure should be used to guide the administration of analgesics.

- Water should be restricted until the animal fully recovers and may be withheld until the following morning. Similarly, withholding food until the next day may be necessary. Consult with the veterinarian regarding these issues.
- Daily monitoring of the patient should continue as long as necessary in order to ensure a full recovery. This should include a vital signs check, assessment of any clinical signs, including any indications of pain or distress, wound care, evaluation of food and water intake, and body weight. Veterinary treatments should be based on these assessments (Figure 4.12).

Stages of Anesthesia

Stage I: voluntary excitement

This stage is the period beginning with the induction of anesthesia until the loss of consciousness. Dogs are commonly disorientated and fearful. Struggling, increased salivation, vocalization, vomiting, or diarrhea may occur. Respiration and heart rate are regular (unless the animal is excited), pupil size is normal, muscle tone is normal, and reflexes are still present. Analgesia is variable but usually limited.

Stage II: involuntary excitement or delirium

This stage is the period when early loss of consciousness occurs. Paradoxically the central nervous system (CNS) appears to be stimulated through selective depression of inhibitory centers in the brain. As voluntary control is lost, dogs may struggle, resulting in injuries. Respirations are generally irregular and breath-holding may occur. Pupil size is dilated, eyes are wide open, muscle tone and reflexes are still present, and increased vocalization, vomiting, or diarrhea may occur. Passing through this stage quickly to prevent injury to the dog is important, but one should use caution and avoid administering anesthetics too fast, thus depressing the respiratory center.

Stage III: surgical anesthesia

This stage is the period when unconsciousness and progressive depression of respiration, circulation, muscle tone, and protective reflexes (eye, pedal, swallowing, gag, etc.) occurs. Pupil size is normal to slightly dilated, muscles are relaxed, and respiration is of a regular rate and depth. Noxious stimuli do not elicit a response.

Post Operative / Post Anesthetic Monitoring Record

Protocol Number _____   Principal Investigator _____   Extension _____   Animal Location _____

Animal ID # _____   Date of Surgery/Anesthesia _____   Procedure _____

Post Operative Monitoring Instructions/Therapeutics: _____

Post Op Day	Temp	HR	RR	CRT	Stools-Urine	Surgical Site	Appetite	Behavior/Attitude	Treatments	Initials
1										
2										
3										
4										
5										
6										
7										
8										
9										
10										

KEY: Temp = Temperature (°F), HR = Heart Rate (beats per minute), RR = Respiratory Rate (beats per minute), CRT = Capillary Refill Time (seconds).

Comments (Specify date for all comments):

Figure 4.12 Postoperative/postanesthetic monitoring record form.

Stage IV: medullary paralysis and respiratory arrest

This stage results when the CNS becomes overly depressed. If immediate resuscitory actions are not undertaken, then respiratory arrest followed by a slowing heart rate and death may occur.[18,19]

Assessment of the Depth of Anesthesia

Respiration

Observation of respiratory patterns should begin prior to induction of anesthesia. Rate, rhythm, and depth are key parameters to note. Assuming normal respiratory patterns to start, as one passes through stage II, irregular patterns begin and panting, hyperventilation, or breath-holding may occur. During stage III, a regular rate and depth and smooth rhythm begins. The surgical plane of anesthesia may straddle a fine line where the respiratory rate and rhythm vary from regular to irregular and the depth of respiration becomes shallower. Abdominal respiration, shallower depth, and an irregular rate occur with an increasing depth of anesthesia. Respiratory rate may increase with extensive surgical manipulations and this does not automatically indicate an inadequate depth of anesthesia.

Cardiovascular

Note the cardiovascular parameters prior to induction. Heart rate, rhythm, pulse, capillary refill time (CRT), and blood pressure are key parameters to note. Heart rate and rhythm progress from a steady rate and rhythm with a strong pulse preinduction to a rapid heart rate and elevated blood pressure during stage II, to a regular heart rate and rhythm (perhaps slightly elevated) during surgical anesthesia (stage III). The pulse should be strong and steady at surgical anesthesia. As the depth of anesthesia progresses deeper, the heart rate will decrease and then weaken and the blood pressure will drop. Surgical manipulations can affect the heart rate. The CRT can be used as a general indicator of circulatory function where one observes a return to normal color of the gums in less than 1.5 seconds after blanching the oral mucosa by gently pressing with a finger.

Reflexes

Laryngeal and pedal reflexes can be monitored as indicators of the depth of anesthesia, and the pedal reflex can also be used to assess the presence of pain. These reflexes are present and exaggerated during stage II and are absent during surgical anesthesia.

Ocular

Eyeball position and movement, pupil size, and palpebral and corneal reflexes are key parameters to monitor. The eyeball progresses from a variable position with a constricted pupil during stage I to centrally fixed and with a dilated pupil with or without nystagmus in stage II. In stage III, the eyeball rotates medially, and the pupil varies from constricted to moderately dilated. As the depth of anesthesia progresses, the eyeball is centrally fixed, and the pupils dilate. The palpebral reflex becomes diminished to absent in surgical anesthesia, and the corneal reflex is absent during deeper anesthesia.

Note: Remember that the effects of anesthesia are variable and an assessment of the depth should account for the variable onset and duration of the selected regimen in the individual patient. The same signs can be used to monitor recovery from anesthesia in reverse order.[18,19]

Preanesthetic Management

Premedication of an animal prior to the induction of general anesthesia is a common and often necessary practice. It contributes to a balanced anesthetic regimen and smoother recovery. Sedatives or tranquilizers are used to decrease fear and anxiety and calm the animal. Anticholinergics are used to decrease oral secretions and gastric motility. Analgesics are used to assist with pain relief intra- and postoperatively. Antibiotics may be administered preoperatively to prevent infections. Eye ointment during or following anesthesia is recommended to prevent drying of the eye.

Veterinarians should be consulted to develop the best preanesthetic and anesthetic regimens for the research project. They can also help assess potential drug interactions in order to minimize potential complications to the research. As previously discussed, one should perform a good physical examination to ensure the animal is in good health and an acceptable candidate for the procedure. During this examination, an accurate body weight should be obtained for dose calculations. Preanesthetic drugs can affect recovery times. Table 4.5 lists typical agents and dosages.

Characteristics of Commonly used Preanesthetics

Some of the characteristics of commonly used preanesthetics are discussed below and are listed in Table 4.5.

- Acepromazine is a phenothiazine tranquilizer helpful to restrain and calm an animal. It also has antiemetic and antispasmodic effects but provides no analgesia.
- Atipamezole is an alpha-2 antagonist used to reverse medetomidine.
- Atropine and glycopyyrolate are anticholinergic drugs administered to decrease salivary, respiratory, and gastric secretions to relax the gastrointestinal tract and prevent a decrease in heart rate. Glycopyyrolate is longer acting than atropine.
- Buprenorphine is an opioid narcotic analgesic that provides long-lasting analgesia.
- Diazepam and midazolam are benzodiazepine tranquilizers that are helpful to restrain and calm an animal. They have muscle relaxation and anticonvulsive effects, but provide no analgesia. Midazolam is two to three times stronger than diazepam, but has a shorter duration of effect.
- Medetomidine is an alpha-2 adrenergic agonist tranquilizer that provides dose-dependent sedation and limited analgesia. It potentiates other anesthetic drugs and is reversible by atipamezole.

Choosing an Anesthetic Regimen

Selection of an anesthetic regimen is based on multiple factors, including the goals of the research, the health status of the patient, the potential for pain and the duration of the procedure, the availability and experience of personnel to assist with anesthesia, and the availability of precision vaporizers and monitoring equipment.

Choosing between gas or injectable anesthetics or combinations of the two is another key consideration. Gas anesthetics generally have a rapid and smooth onset and are quickly eliminated by the lungs, permitting careful control of the depth of anesthesia. They require expensive precision vaporizers, systems to scavenge waste gases to prevent human exposure, and personnel to run and monitor anesthesia.

Injectable anesthetics require minimal equipment and have a quick onset, which safeguards both personnel and the patient, especially when animals struggle. The depth of anesthesia is harder to control, and the more extensive biotransformation process required to eliminate injectables prolongs recovery. Using injectables as part of the preanesthetic induction regimen followed by maintenance with gas anesthesia is a common practice and provides for a balanced anesthetic regimen with quick recovery. Consultation with a veterinarian is recommended to determine an appropriate anesthetic regimen.

Characteristics of Commonly Used Injectable Anesthetics

Some of the characteristics of commonly used injectable anesthetics are discussed below and are listed in Table 4.6.

Propofol is a newer alkyl phenol anesthetic agent that can be used for the induction and maintenance of short and long anesthetic procedures or can be used as part of a balanced anesthetic regimen. It has rapid onset and recovery and good control of the depth of anesthesia. Induction is by slow infusion over about 10 to 20 seconds, and maintenance of anesthesia is by continuous infusion or incremental dosing. Dose-dependent cardiopulmonary and CNS depression may be seen, and apnea may occur during induction. Transient pain on injection may be seen.

Thiopental is an ultra-short-acting barbiturate that can be used as an anesthetic agent for radiographs, examinations, short surgical procedures, or as an induction agent prior to an inhalant anesthetic. Repeat administration provides extended anesthesia. In dogs, it can cause arrhythmia, tachycardia, and respiratory depression. Inadvertent administration of intravenous doses into subcutaneous tissues will cause necrosis.

Pentobarbital is an intermediate-acting barbiturate that is commonly used as an anesthetic agent for surgical procedures. When used as the sole anesthetic agent, it is recommended that one administer about half of the calculated dose initially and the rest to effect. Surgical anesthesia occurs at doses close to those causing respiratory failure and cardiovascular depression. Phenothiazine tranquilizers or opioid analgesics are used to minimize difficult recoveries common with pentobarbital, where dogs will vocalize or thrash around.

principles of gas anesthesia

The use of gas anesthetic agents requires precision vaporizers, scavenging systems for removal of waste anesthetic gases in order to prevent personnel exposure, endotracheal intubation (preferably versus the use of a face mask or nose cone) to deliver anesthesia to the animal, and trained and experienced staff familiar with the use of the anesthetic equipment for induction and monitoring of anesthesia. Prior to use, anesthesia machines should be inspected to ensure they are in working order, that there is sufficient anesthetic agent for the procedure, and that the soda lime canister has a usable quantity remaining.[18-22]

Characteristics of Commonly Used Gas Anesthetics

Some of the characteristics of commonly used gas anesthetics are discussed below.

Isoflurane is a commonly used agent for providing general anesthesia in the dog. It provides fast and smooth induction and recovery, good control of the depth of anesthesia, excellent muscle relaxation, has minimal cardiovascular depression at surgical anesthesia, and does not sensitize the heart to the effect of catecholamines, which can lead to arrhythmia. It requires a precision vaporizer.

Sevoflurane is a less frequently used inhalant anesthetic for dogs. Its odor is less offensive than isoflurane, so dogs are less likely to hold their breath during induction by gas inhalation. It tends to be more expensive that isoflurane and it also requires a precision vaporizer.

Halothane is a general anesthetic agent used in the dog. It provides rapid induction and recovery, albeit longer than with isoflurane, good muscle relaxation, moderate cardiopulmonary depression, and sensitization of the heart to catecholamines. It requires a precision vaporizer and is expensive. The availability of halothane is diminishing because of the popularity of other anesthetics.

Nitrous oxide is generally used as an adjunctive agent with other narcotic or gas anesthetic agents in order to reduce their adverse effects. It enhances the uptake of other gas anesthetics, provides supplemental analgesia, and has minimal cardiopulmonary depression. Nitrous oxide should be discontinued about 5 minutes before oxygen is discontinued to prevent diffusion hypoxia.

principles of local anesthesia

The use of local anesthesia in research settings is uncommon, as preference is given to the use of general anesthetics. When general anesthesia is not desired, local anesthesia can be used for minor procedures such as small skin biopsies. It can also be used to prevent laryngospasm during intubation. Local anesthesia is useful in combination with a sedative when additional restraint is required, or as supplement to general anesthesia for additional analgesia around the incision site. Commonly used local anesthetics include lidocaine or the longer-acting bupivicaine.[21]

aseptic surgery

Asepsis is the absence of pathologic organisms in living tissues. Sterilization is the process of killing all microorganisms with either physical or chemical agents. Aseptic surgery involves preventing contamination of tissues by microbes. Survival surgery in dogs must be performed in a surgical suite employing aseptic technique in order to reduce microbial contamination of the animal. Aseptic surgery includes the following:

- Patient preparation includes clipping or shaving of the hair, disinfection of the skin, and draping the surgical site with sterile drapes.
- Surgeon preparation includes performing a surgical scrub of the hands and forearms, and donning a sterilized gown over scrubs, sterile gloves, a surgical mask, and hair bonnet.
- Instrument preparation involves sterilization of all instruments, supplies, and implantable items such as sutures and catheters.
- Good operative technique is designed to reduce the risk of contamination and infection of the surgical site, ensure gentle handling of tissues to minimize trauma, and prevent blood loss by providing good hemostasis.

Facilities, Features, and Equipment

Regulations require that survival surgery performed in dogs occur in a surgical facility. The *Guide* lists the following key functional areas of a surgical facility: surgical support, animal preparation, surgeon's scrub room, operating room, and postoperative recovery areas (Figure 4.13). Separation of these areas by physical barriers is preferred over separation by distance.[22]

In order to reduce the risk of contamination, the surgical facility should be constructed of impervious surfaces that are easily disinfected and sanitized. It should have positive pressure in the operating room versus other rooms in the suite. The operating room and surrounding area should be restricted to surgical personnel only during the procedure in order to maintain aseptic technique. Other important features include the following:

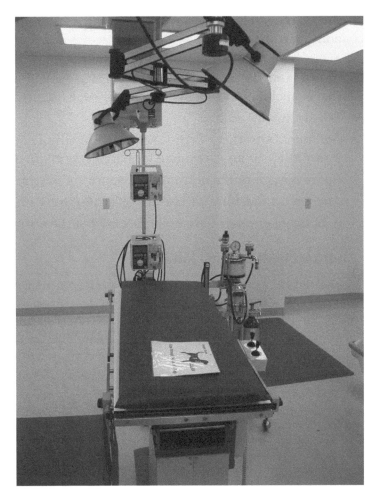

Figure 4.13 Operating room with good lighting, anesthesia machine, and patient monitoring equipment.

- Surgical lights that illuminate the surgical area.
- A circulating warm-water heating pad to maintain body temperature.
- An adjustable height operating table.
- Various surgical packs appropriate for the planned procedures and additional equipment as needed.
- Autoclave, cold sterilant solutions, or glass bead sterilizer. Cold sterilants should be rinsed with sterile saline prior to use in animals. Instruments should be cleaned of debris and rinsed with sterile saline before placing in a glass bead sterilizer.

- Intravenous solutions, stands, warming units, and pumps for fluid administration.
- A variety of equipment is helpful for monitoring patients while under anesthesia, including an EKG, pulse oximeter, rectal thermometer, and esophageal stethoscope (Figure 4.14).
- Trash cans for waste.
- Additional anesthetic drugs, a crash cart with emergency drugs, and a respirator or an Ambu bag for patient ventilation (Figure 4.15).
- Spare oxygen tanks or an in-line source of oxygen.
- Anesthesia machine with scavenging (Figure 4.16).
- A footstool or chair for ergonomic relief of the surgeon(s).

Endotracheal Intubation

Endotracheal tube placement is the preferred method of delivering gas anesthesia to and removing waste gases from a patient, especially for longer anesthetic procedures. Tubes should be selected to best match the size of the animal's airway. Sizes range from 4 to 12 mm inside diameter (ID) for small to medium size dogs and 12 to 18 mm ID for medium to large dogs (Figure 4.17). Tubes should be

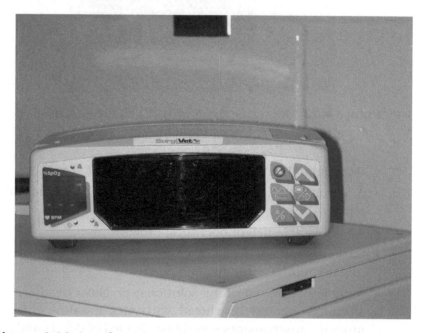

Figure 4.14 A pulse oximeter is used to monitor a patient during anesthesia or surgery.

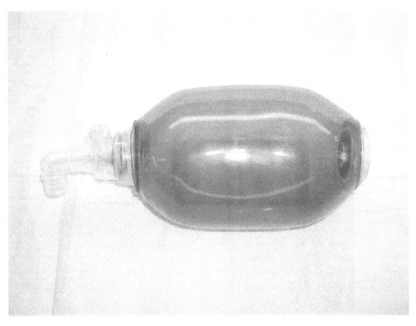

Figure 4.15 An Ambu bag is used to manually ventilate a patient.

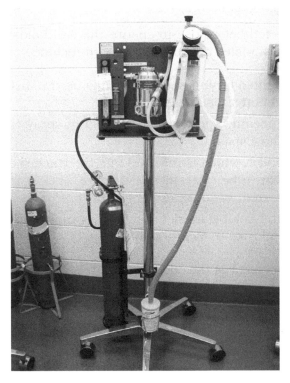

Figure 4.16 A portable anesthesia machine.

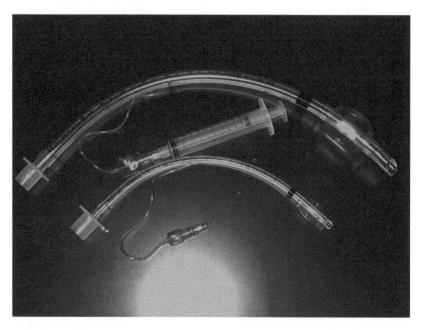

Figure 4.17 Endotracheal tubes should be selected to easily pass into the trachea. Gently inflating the cuff "snugs" the tube in place.

inspected before use to ensure the cuff holds air without deflating. Other supplies that may be needed include

- A lighted laryngoscope, which is used to help deflect the epiglottis and better visualize the airway.
- Lignocaine spray, which is used to spray the larynx and prevent laryngospasm.
- A stylet, which is inserted into the trachea as a guide for endotracheal tube placement. Remove the stylet after the tube is inserted.
- Water-soluble lubricant, which is applied to the tip of the endotracheal tube to facilitate insertion.

Placement of the endotracheal tube is as follows:

1   Anesthetize and place the dog in sternal recumbency.
2.   Open the mouth and pull the tongue forward and down. Use a gauze pad for a better grip on the tongue.
3.   Place the endotracheal tube over the tongue and into the back of the oral cavity. The tip of the tube can be used to deflect the epiglottis if a laryngoscope is not used.

4. Pause until the dog takes a breath, which dilates the opening to the trachea. Pass the endotracheal tube into the trachea and advance it into position.

5. After placement in the trachea, the cuff should be gently inflated to prevent leakage around the tube.

6. Verify tube placement in the trachea by observing the passage of air. The tube should slightly fog up or deflect a tissue placed at the tube opening.

7. Secure the tube to the muzzle using a gauze tie. Tie the gauze around the endotracheal tube and then around the muzzle. This will prevent dislodging of the tube.

8. Connect the anesthesia machine to the tube.

Tubes should be cleaned and disinfected after use and should be stored properly between uses. Face masks and nose cones are alternatives to this method and these should fit snugly over the snout to minimize dead space.

Personnel

The availability of an adequate number of personnel trained and experienced to conduct the procedure is essential. In addition to the **surgeon**, an **assistant** is needed for patient preparation, anesthesia induction and monitoring, and for general support of the surgeon. A **surgical assistant** may be needed to directly assist the surgeon with the procedure. Operating room personnel should wear surgical scrubs and put on surgical masks and hair bonnets prior to scrubbing for surgery. Surgeons and assistant surgeons must wear sterile gowns and gloves. Operating room assistants need not wear sterile gowns and gloves, but clean surgical scrubs with or without clean lab coats should be worn.

Preoperative Preparation

As discussed previously, perform a clinical examination and obtain a body weight to determine the doses of anesthetics. Moving the animal to a quiet area prior to anesthesia is recommended.

Premedicate the animal with atropine, acepromazine, antibiotics, or other medications about 30 minutes prior to anesthesia induction.

Clip an area on the foreleg and place a catheter for use in administration of intravenous anesthetics (especially barbiturates), fluids during surgery, and any emergency drugs.

Induce anesthesia and place and secure the endotracheal tube. Clip or shave the surgical site and perform a preliminary surgical scrub of the area.

Connect intravenous fluids and patient monitoring devices such as an EKG.

Transfer the animal to the operating room and place it on the operating table outfitted with a circulating warm-water heating pad and complete the surgical scrub of the dog. This involves performing three alternating scrubs using an antiseptic scrub (e.g., betadine or chlorhexidine) followed by 70% alcohol. Starting at the center of the incision site, move outward in a circular manner. Scrub sponges should be discarded after one pass.

Concurrent with patient preparation, the surgeon and assistant surgeon should remove any jewelry and perform a surgical scrub in order to maintain surgical asepsis. This involves cleaning under fingernails and then, while keeping hands held vertical, performing three timed scrubs, working from the fingertips to the elbows, using a surgical scrub. Each hand is done in alternating fashion, and the lather should be left on one arm while scrubbing the other to increase contact time. Rinse and dry each arm after the final scrub.

Assistants should help the surgeon(s) with donning a sterile gown and gloves. Gowns are considered sterile from the top of the surgical table to chest height. Caution must be used to not lower hands below this level to prevent breaking with aseptic technique. Similarly, gloves must be changed when punctured or contaminated, as failure to do so risks contamination of the animal and infection.

The surgeon should drape the dog before starting the procedure. A final check to verify the proper depth of anesthesia should be performed before making the first incision.

Operating Room Procedures

The operating room and surrounding area should be restricted to surgical personnel only during the procedure in order to maintain aseptic technique. Standard surgical techniques should be employed, including the use of appropriate surgical tools to manipulate tissues, gentle handling of all tissues, prevention of blood loss, keeping tissues moist, and the use of appropriate needles and suture material for the tissues.

postsurgical management

This begins immediately following completion of the procedure, when the animal is still anesthetized, and extends until full recovery of the animal and removal of the sutures. Often, animals will have procedures performed as part of study initiation shortly after surgery, so sutures may not be removed before a study begins.

During the immediate postoperative period until the animal is awake and has achieved sternal recumbency, the animal should have frequent monitoring of vital signs (TPR and pain) and the incision site. Discontinue anesthesia and maintain the animal on oxygen, especially if nitrous oxide was used. Maintain supplemental heat through use of a heating pad and a drape. Remove the endotracheal tube when the animal is awake and swallowing and gag reflexes are normal, as indicated by regular chewing motions. Fluids can be discontinued, but the catheter should be maintained. Transfer the animal to a heated recovery cage after removal of the endotracheal tube and cover it with a blanket. The animal will move out from under the blanket when it has recovered and is at a normal body temperature. Administer analgesics and other medications based on patient evaluations in consultation with a veterinarian. Withholding water and food is necessary until the swallowing reflex is normal and the animal is fully awake. In some cases, food and water are withheld until the following morning. Controlled amounts of water can be administered using a syringe. Records of all postoperative care should be accurately maintained.

The day after surgery, regular monitoring of vital signs and the incision site should continue throughout the day, with medications being administered as needed. The incision site should be checked for problems such as dried blood, exudates, inflammation, or dehiscence. It should be cleaned regularly with sterile saline and antiseptic. Bandages should be used when needed and changed regularly. Water can be offered *ad libitum*, but return the animal to food at half its normal ration, providing smaller amounts regularly throughout the day. The animal can be transferred to its normal cage when released by the veterinarian.

In subsequent days, monitoring frequency can be tapered off based on clinical assessment, and food can be returned to normal quantities. Sutures should be removed at 10 to 14 days after surgery. Document clinical assessments and treatments thoroughly and maintain these as part of the animal's permanent record.

guidelines for the assessment of signs of pain in animals

These guidelines are provided for use as general indicators of pain or discomfort. They cover a variety of parameters that can be used to assess an animal's health status and guide veterinary care. Interpretation of the signs to assess clinical status and treatment plans should be performed under the direction of a veterinarian.

- Activity: Decreased food and water intake, reflex withdrawal, biting at the source of pain or affected area, increased activity, aversive behavior toward cage mates.
- Appearance: Piloerection, weight loss, sunken abdomen, or dehydration.
- Defecation: Constipation, impaction, or diarrhea.
- Eyes: Sunken with or without discharge or almost closed.
- General: Hypothermia, hyperthermia, or weight loss.
- Locomotion: Stilted gait or lameness.
- Posture: Recumbent, hunched, hunched with head tucked into abdomen, standing with front legs apart, or "sleeping" posture.
- Respiration: Increased respiratory rate, labored breathing, "chattering," or nasal discharge.
- Restlessness: Shaking or scratching a particular area, hyperactive, or circling.
- Self-mutilation: Excessive licking or chewing of an appendage.
- Temperament: More or less docile or aggressive, quiet, unsociable, or depressed, leading to unresponsiveness.
- Urination: Increased or decreased urination or incontinence.
- Vocalization: Squeals, moans, whines, or barks on handling or when pressure is exerted on the affected area.

blood donors

The need for replacement of whole blood or blood components (e.g., thrombocytes) may arise. Commercial blood banks are available for these purposes in the United States and Canada, but the availability of onsite donor animals provides a more immediate option. Typing and cross matching is recommended to avoid transfusion reactions and to prevent sensitization of the recipient to future transfusions.

Donors should be free of blood-borne pathogens (e.g., heartworm and *Ehrlichia*) and 20 μm millipore filters are recommended to filter out potential platelet aggregations. Additional sources should be consulted for more details.[25-26]

euthanasia

Euthanasia refers to the act of inducing a humane death in animals. It should be conducted in a manner that is as painless and stress free as possible for the animal. Due consideration should also be given to the human behavioral elements associated with performing canine euthanasia where emotional attachments may be present. It is important, when assigning this to an individual, to seek assurance that they are comfortable with performing the procedure.

Euthanasia should be performed by an approved method according to study-specific endpoint criteria as described in the protocol. Signs of illness or disease and selected criteria for animal euthanasia are provided as general references to help assess the clinical condition of the animal and determine its prognosis.

signs of morbidity (state of disease or illness) in animals

Signs of morbidity include the following:

- Rapid respiratory rate.
- Slow, shallow, labored breathing.
- Hunched posture.
- Ruffled fur (rough hair coat).
- Hyper- or hypothermia.
- Rapid weight loss (20% to 25% of normal body weight within 1 to 2 weeks).
- Diarrhea, vomiting, or constipation.
- Prolonged loss of appetite or cachexia.
- Behavioral changes.
- Skin sores, ulcerative dermatitis, or infections.
- Decreased activity.
- Inability to obtain food or water.
- Ocular discharge.

selected criteria for euthanasia of moribund (state of dying) animals

Criteria for euthanasia of moribund animals includes the following:

- Rapid weight loss (15% to 25% in 1 week).
- Extended period of weight loss progressing to emaciation.
- Rough hair coat, hunched posture, distended abdomen, or lethargy, especially if debilitating or prolonged (more than 3 days).
- Diarrhea or vomiting, especially if debilitating or prolonged (more than 3 days).
- Persistent cough, rales, wheezing, nasal discharge, or respiratory distress.
- Distinct icterus.
- Persistent anemia leading to debilitation.
- Central nervous system signs such as head tilt, tremors, spasticity, seizures, circling, or paresis, especially if associated with anorexia.
- Persistent bleeding from any orifice.
- Paralysis.
- Markedly discolored urine, polyuria, or anuria especially if pro longed (more than 3 days).
- Persistent self-induced trauma.
- Impaired mobility or lesions interfering with eating or drinking.
- Clinical signs of suspected infectious disease requiring a necropsy for diagnosis.
- Other clinical signs judged by experienced technical staff to be indicative of a moribund condition.
- Cyanosis.

The most common methods used to euthanize dogs are an overdose with a barbiturate or inhalant anesthetic. Premedication with a tranquilizer prior to barbiturate overdose is another consideration for aggressive animals. In all cases, death must be ensured and verified. Some institutions require a secondary means of ensuring euthanasia, such as opening the chest cavity (pneumothorax), which collapses the lungs. Refer to the 2000 report of the American Veterinary Medical Association Panel on Euthanasia for additional details.[27]

references

1. Dysko, R.C., Nemzek, J.A., Levin, S.I., DeMarco, G.J., and Moalli, M.R., Biology and diseases of dogs, in *Laboratory Animal Medicine*, 2nd ed., Fox, J.G., Anderson, L.C., Loew, F.M., and Quimby, F.W., eds., Academic Press, San Diego, 2002, chap. 11.

2. Kahn, C.M. and Line, S., eds., *The Merck Veterinary Manual*, 9th ed., Merck & Co., Whitehouse Station, NJ, 2005.

3. Greene, C.E., ed., *Clinical Microbiology and Infectious Diseases of the Dog and Cat*, W.B. Saunders, Philadelphia, 1984.

4. Greene, C.E., editor, *Infectious Diseases of the Dog and Cat*, 2nd ed., W.B. Saunders, Philadelphia, 1998.

5. Kovacs, M.S., McKiernan, S., Poptter, D.M., and Shilappagari, S., An epidemiological study of interdigital cysts in a research beagle colony, *Contemp. Top. Lab. Anim. Sci.*, 44(4), 17, 2005.

6. Hayes, T.J., Roberts, G.K., and Halliwell, W.H., An idiopathic febrile necrotizing arteritis syndrome in the dog: beagle pain syndrome, *Toxicol. Pathol.*, 17(1 pt. 2), 129, 1989.

7. Albassam, M.A., Houston, B.J., Greaves, P., and Barsoum, N., Polyarteritis in a beagle, *J. Am. Vet. Med. Assoc.*, 194, 1595, 1989.

8. Son, W.C., Idiopathic canine polyarteritis in control beagles from toxicity studies, *J. Vet. Sci.*, 5, 147, 2004.

9. Slatter, D.H., Nictitating membrane, in *Fundamentals of Veterinary Ophthalmology*, W.B. Saunders, Philadelphia, 1981, chap. 9.

10. Moore, C.P., Third eyelid, in *Textbook of Small Animal Surgery*, 2nd ed., Slatter, D., ed., W.B. Saunders, Philadelphia, 1993, chap. 85.

11. Frost, P., *Canine Dentistry: A Compendium*, 2nd ed., Day Communications, Mount Kisco, NY, 1985.

12. Dorn, A.S., Dentistry, in *Textbook of Small Animal Surgery*, 2nd ed., Slatter, D., ed., W.B. Saunders, Philadelphia, 1993, chap. 175.

13. Dorsten, C.M. and Cooper, D.M., Use of body condition scoring to manage body weights in dogs, *Contemp. Top. Lab. Anim. Sci.*, 43(3), 34, 2004.

14. DiBartola, S.P., Gastrointestinal Problems, in *Quick Reference to Veterinary Medicine*, Fenner, W.R., ed., J.B. Lippincott Co., Philadelphia, 1982.

15. Kirk, R.W. and Bistner, S.I, eds., Interpreting signs of disease, in *Handbook of Veterinary Procedures and Emergency Treatment*, 4th ed., W.B. Saunders, Philadelphia, 1985.

16. Allen, D.G., Pringle, J.K., and Smith, D., eds., *Handbook of Veterinary Drugs*, J.B. Lippincott, Philadelphia, 1993.

17. Smith, B.P., House, J.K., Magdesian, K.G., Jang, S.S., Cabral R.L. Jr., Madigan, J.E., and Herthel, W.F., Principles of an infectious disease control program for preventing nosocomial gastrointestinal and respiratory diseases in large animal veterinary hospitals, *J. Am. Vet. Med. Assoc.*, 225, 1186, 2004.

18. Hubbell, J.A.E. and Muir, W.W., eds., *Handbook of Veterinary Anesthesia*, C.V. Mosby, St. Louis, 1989.

19. Slatter, D., ed., *Textbook of Small Animal Surgery*, 2nd ed., W.B. Saunders, Philadelphia, 1993.

20. Flecknell, P.A., *Laboratory Animal Anesthesia*, Academic Press, San Diego, 1987.

21. Flecknell, P.A., *Laboratory Animal Anesthesia*, 2nd ed., Academic Press, San Diego, 1996.

22. Kohn, D.F., Wixson, S.K., White, W.J., and Benson, G.J., eds., *Anesthesia and Analgesia in Laboratory Animals*, Academic Press, San Diego, 1997.

23. Hawk, C.T. and Leary, S.L., eds., *Formulary for Laboratory Animals*, Iowa State University Press, Ames, 1995.

24. Hawk, C.T. and Leary, S.L., eds., *Formulary for Laboratory Animals*, 2nd ed., Iowa State University Press, Ames, 1999.

25. Dodds, W.J., Canine and feline blood groups, in *Textbook of Small Animal Surgery*, Slatter, D.H., ed., W.B. Saunders, Philadelphia, 1985.

26. Baldwin, C.J., Cowell, R.L., Kostolich, M., Tyler, R.D., and Sempere, D.C., Hemostasis: physiology, diagnosis, and treatment of bleeding disorders in surgical patients, in *Textbook of Small Animal Surgery*, 2nd ed., Slatter, D., ed., W.B. Saunders, Philadelphia, 1993, p. 29.

27. AVMA Panel on Euthanasia, American Veterinary Medical Association, 2000 Report of the AVMA Panel on Euthanasia, *J. Am. Vet. Med. Assoc.*, 218, 669, 2001.

28. Booth, N.H., *Veterinary Pharmacology and Therapeutics*, 5th ed., Booth, N.H. and McDonald, L.E., eds., Iowa State University Press, Ames, 1982, chap. 16.

experimental methodology

Dogs are commonly used in a wide variety of animal research, including surgical models, routine pharmacology and toxicology testing, and teaching. A comprehensive list of all procedures performed on dogs is beyond the scope of this book, but the most common procedures will be described.

canine handling and restraint

Manual restraint of most laboratory dogs is best accomplished with gentle handling and acclimation to the restraint prior to the start of the experiment. Most dogs react well to a soft, calming voice speaking to them during the restraint. Fractious animals that need stronger restraint or sedation to keep them from biting or scratching personnel should not be used in research.

For manual restraint during many procedures, the dog is placed on an examining table. The dog is given a gentle "hug" with one arm under the neck to control the head and the other arm gently holding the rest of the body. If drawing blood or injecting into a cephalic vein, the second arm can be used to occlude the vein at the elbow. Hyperactive or highly energetic animals may be briefly restrained by using the second hand to grasp the skin at the scruff (back) of the neck (Figure 5.1).

For fractious animals that must be handled, various size muzzles are commercially available. If a manufactured muzzle is unavailable, a suitable substitute can be made out of a piece of strong gauze. A loop with a half hitch at the top is placed over the dog's nose and mouth. The loop is tightened, and the ends are brought down to tie another half hitch under the muzzle. From there, the ends are

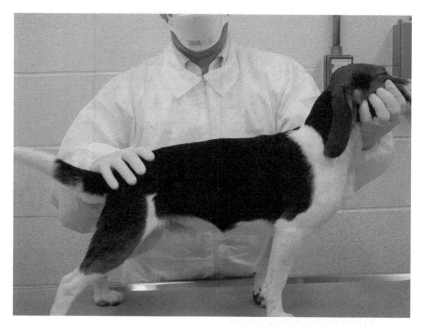

(a)

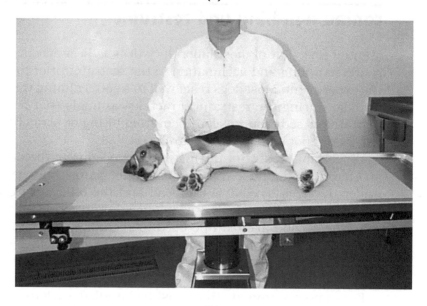

(b)

Figure 5.1 Dog restraint: (a) standing restraint for a physical exam and (b) lateral restraint for an electrocardiogram (EKG) or other procedure.

brought behind the neck at the level of the ears to tie another half hitch and then a bowknot.

Mechanical Restraint Devices

Some examination tables come equipped with a vertical arm and a rope leash to fit over the dog's neck. These are often used by pet groomers and are suitable for keeping reasonably cooperative animals on the table and facing in one direction without the assistance of a second individual. These dogs should not be left unattended. Slings are also commercially available to restrain dogs without the need for an assistant (Figure 5.2). The length of time a dog is restrained should be minimized, and any prolonged restraint should be approved by the Institutional Animal Care and Use Committee (IACUC). Acclimating dogs to manual restraint devices prior to study initiation is recommended.

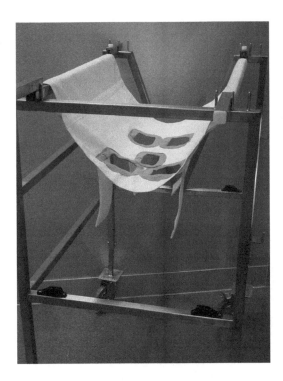

Figure 5.2 Dog sling for restraint.

sample collection methods

Blood Collection

Blood may be collected from jugular veins, cephalic veins, and lateral saphenous veins in the dog. Although typically avoided in pet dogs for cosmetic reasons, hair may be clipped from over the vein in laboratory dogs to improve visualization. Before inserting the needle, the skin may be swabbed with 70% alcohol or another suitable antiseptic.

Various types of collection containers can be used, depending on the skill and preference of the collector. Often blood is collected in a syringe to allow the collector to control the amount of negative pressure used and to avoid collapsing the vein. Vacutainer tubes may be used with larger veins to minimize hemolysis and to avoid the potential for blood clots forming in the syringe. Generally, red-top tubes (no additive) are used when serum is needed, and purple-top tubes (ethylenediaminetetraacetic acid [EDTA]) are used to collect whole blood for hematology (Figure 5.3).

The blood volume of healthy dogs is approximately 85 ml/kg. Leaner dogs have a higher blood volume per kilogram than obese

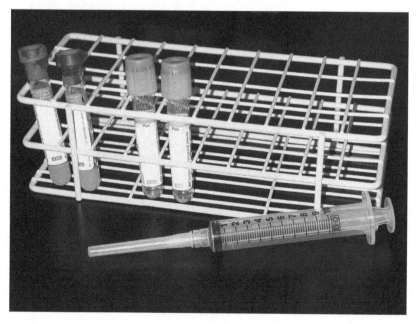

Figure 5.3 Vacutainer tubes used for blood samples collected to analyze hematology (purple top) and clinical chemistry (red top) parameters.

animals. To avoid stress from hypovolemia (excessive blood loss), no more than 10% to 15% of the circulating blood volume should be removed in a single sampling, and no more than 15% to 20% of the circulating blood volume should be removed in a 24 hour period. If more blood is needed, the animal should receive supplemental fluids or transfused blood to prevent hypovolemia. After collections of 7.5% of a dog's blood volume, they should be given a week to recover before more blood is removed. Two weeks are needed to recover from removal of 10% of the blood volume, and three or more weeks are needed for 15% removal.[1]

The jugular vein is the preferred site for blood collection in the dog. Jugular veins are large, easily visualized, and not often used for injections. The dog is restrained in a seated position and the head is gently tilted upward by an assistant. The collector occludes a jugular vein by pressing on the base of the neck to one side. The vein may then be visualized or palpated along the side of the neck. In some animals, the vein may be confused with a neck muscle on palpation. To differentiate between the two, palpate the suspect vein or muscle while releasing the pressure occluding the vein. If the structure in question is the jugular vein, it disappears when pressure is released and returns when the vein is occluded again. If the structure in question was a muscle, it remains visible when pressure is released. Generally, 20- to 22-gauge needles are used for collection (Figure 5.4).

The cephalic veins are the next most commonly used veins for blood collection. They are easily visualized and suitable for collecting small to medium-size samples. The cephalic veins run the length of the forearm from the elbow to the carpus. An assistant restrains the animal with one arm under the neck and another arm holding the dog's leg at the elbow (Figure 5.5). The assistant's thumb is used to occlude the vein and turn it laterally to minimize rolling. Generally 21- to 22-gauge needles are attached to a syringe for collection. Vacutainer tubes are not used, as they often collapse the vein.

The saphenous veins travel across the lateral aspect of the back legs just above the hock. They can be easily visualized after placing occlusive pressure at or just distal to the knee. They are similar in size to the cephalic veins and often are even easier to visualize. Needles are more easily inserted into the cephalic veins, however, because they run in more of a straight line than the saphenous veins. Like the cephalic veins, the saphenous veins are suitable for collecting small to medium-size samples using a syringe with a 21- or 22-gauge needle.

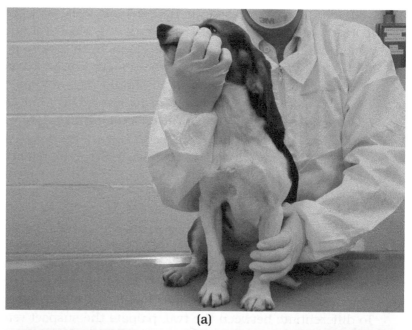

(a)

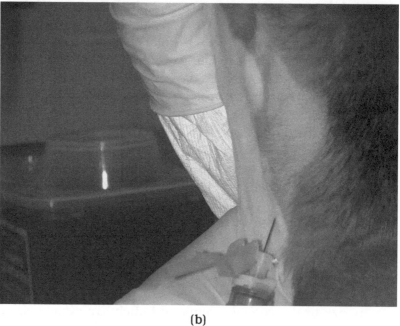

(b)

Figure 5.4 (a) Dog shaved and restrained for jugular blood collection. (b) The jugular vein bulges when occluded during sample collection.

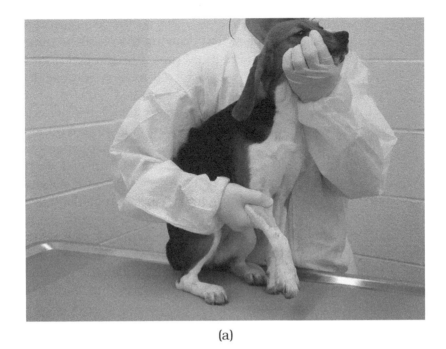

(a)

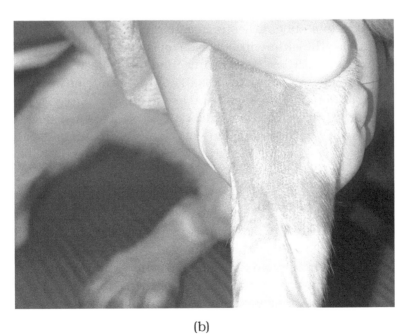

(b)

Figure 5.5 (a) Hug restraint for cephalic blood collection. (b) Prominent cephalic vein.

Regardless of the vein used, the occlusive pressure on the vein should be released before withdrawing the needle to minimize hematoma formation. Gentle manual pressure should be placed over the area where the needle was inserted to stop the bleeding. Alternatively, a temporary bandage can be applied.

If multiple samples are to be collected over a period of a day or two, a catheter should be placed to avoid having to puncture the vein multiple times. The jugular, cephalic, and saphenous veins can all be catheterized. The area over the catheter insertion site is clipped and aseptically scrubbed as for surgery. The vein is occluded and the catheter is inserted pointing in the direction of blood flow. The stylet is removed, the catheter is capped, and it is bandaged in place. The catheter should be flushed with heparinized saline after insertion and periodically thereafter to prevent clotting. When drawing blood, the first 0.5 to 1 ml is discarded before collecting the sample to avoid dilution from the heparinized saline. Indwelling catheters can be left in place for 2 to 3 days.

When multiple samples need to be collected over longer periods of time, vascular access ports (VAPs) are preferred. VAPs are placed surgically into the femoral or jugular veins and tunneled under the skin to a subcutaneous injection port. By keeping the entire system under the skin without external penetration, it can be left in place longer with less risk of infection. To collect a sample or inject the system with heparinized saline to prevent clotting, the area over the injection port is clipped and aseptically prepared as for surgery. Non-coring Huber point needles are used to penetrate the access port. As with catheters, when collecting samples, the first 0.5 to 1 ml of blood is discarded to avoid sample dilution with heparinized saline (Figure 5.6).

Urine Collection

Unlike pet dogs, laboratory dogs are rarely housebroken. It is not practical to follow them on a "walk" to collect a free-catch urine sample. Other methods of urine collection are needed.

The most common method of urine collection in laboratory dogs is the use of metabolism cages. Troughs under the cage funnel the urine to a collection container. As dogs are often left in these cages overnight, the collection containers may be refrigerated to minimize sample deterioration. Some caging manufacturers make pans that fit under run flooring to turn the run into a type of metabolism cage. This prevents the need to purchase and store separate cages for urine

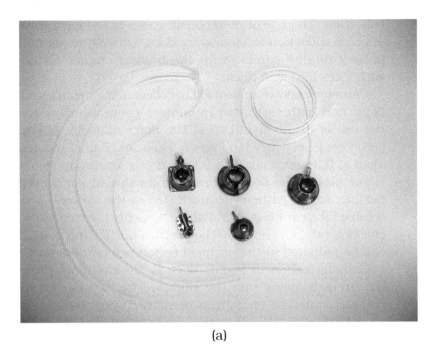

(a)

(b)

Figure 5.6 (a) Vascular access ports (VAPs) and catheters are implanted subcutaneously for long-term access to blood vessels for test article delivery or collection of blood. VAPs are also commonly used for bile collection. (b) Noncoring Huber point needles are recommended for use with access VAPs.

collection. The use of metabolism cages is the least invasive method of urine collection in laboratory dogs. Unfortunately it also gives the poorest quality sample with the highest chance for contamination with feces and feed fines.

Catheterization can be used to collect urine in both male and female dogs, and catheterization minimizes contamination compared with the use of metabolism cages. The outer diameter of canine urinary catheters is measured in French (Fr) units. Each French unit is equivalent to 0.3 mm, making a 9 Fr catheter's outer diameter 3 mm.

For males, the dog is placed on its side in lateral recumbency. A flexible, sterile catheter is lubricated at the tip with a sterile, water-soluble lubricant (e.g., K-Y Jelly). The penis is extruded, and the catheter is gently advanced up the urethra until urine flows. The catheter can be palpated in the perineal region before it enters the bladder.

Catheterization of female dogs is slightly more difficult because the urethra opens into the vagina. The location for insertion of a catheter must be visualized or manually palpated. During digital palpation, a sterile surgical glove is worn and the tip of the finger is lubricated with a sterile, water-soluble lubricant. The urethral papilla is palpated while a sterile catheter is gently fed along the floor of the vagina into the urethral opening at the base of the papilla. To visualize the urethral opening, a vaginal speculum is lubricated and passed into the vagina past the urethral papilla. The handle is gently squeezed to spread the speculum apart to allow visualization. If a vaginal speculum is not available, an otoscope cone can be used with the catheter passed through the cone as the urethral opening is visualized. The catheter is gently passed through the urethral opening until urine is collected. Both flexible and rigid catheters can be used in female dogs.

Catheters may be left in both male and female dogs to collect urine over a period of time. In this case, the use of a closed collection system is preferred to prevent the retrograde introduction of bacteria up the catheter into the bladder. To prepare a closed collection system, tubing used for intravenous fluid administration is connected to the catheter. The other end of the tubing is connected to a collection bag. Urine flows from the catheter into the bag continuously. When closed collection systems are used, the dog must be prevented from chewing on the tubing, often with the use of an Elizabethan collar.

Urine is readily aspirated directly from the bladder of both male and female dogs by cystocentesis. The procedure causes minimal pain and distress, is simple and fast, and produces the best quality, sterile urine samples. For average-size dogs, a 12 ml syringe is connected to a 1½ in., 22-gauge needle. One or more assistants restrain the dog on its back in dorsal recumbency and **the area is aseptically prepared.** In female dogs, the needle is inserted on the midline, just cranial to the pubis, pointed caudally, at a 45-degree angle to the body wall (Figure 5.7). In males, the needle is inserted to the side of the penis and angled toward the midline. Once inserted, urine is aspirated directly into a syringe.

Cerebrospinal Fluid Collection

To collect cerebrospinal fluid (CSF) in dogs, **general anesthesia and aseptic technique are required.** The dog is placed on its side in lateral recumbency and the back of the head and neck are clipped and scrubbed as for surgery and sterile surgical gloves are worn. While the head is held at a right angle to the vertebral column, a sterile spinal needle with a stylet (usually 22-gauge, 1½ in.) is passed between the atlas (first cervical vertebrae) and the occipital bone on

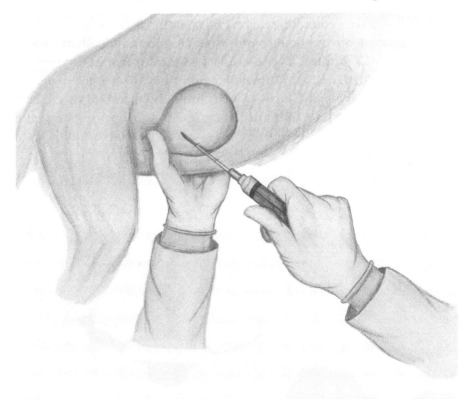

Figure 5.7 Conscious dog in lateral recumbency for collection of urine by cystocentesis. (Courtesy of Jodi Carlson, Yale University)

the back of the head. Care should be taken not to occlude the airway while positioning the head and neck. As the needle punctures the dura matter, a popping sensation is felt. If the dog is only lightly anesthetized, muscle tremors may be seen. At that point the stylet is removed to allow the flow of CSF. CSF should be allowed to drip into the collection container rather than applying negative pressure by syringe (Figure 5.8). CSF may be analyzed for cellular, biochemical, or drug content.

Collection of Feces

The most common reason for collecting feces is to obtain a sample for parasitology. Usually, fresh feces is collected from the cage or run before cleaning. If there is no feces present in the cage or run or if a fresher sample is needed, a fecal collection loop can be used. The loop is lubricated with a water-soluble lubricant and inserted into the anus. The loop is then rotated gently to collect feces before being removed.

Another common reason for collecting feces is to analyze it for drug content during adsorption, distribution, metabolism, and excretion (ADME) studies. These studies require testing of various body fluids (blood, CSF, and urine) or excretions (feces) for drugs of interest and their metabolites. Most commonly, metabolism cages are used for this purpose. Because experimental drugs are often labeled with radioisotopes during ADME studies, special handling procedures

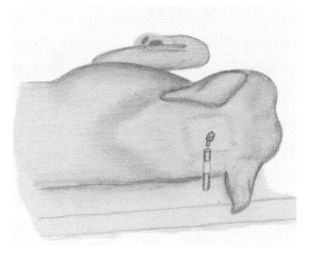

Figure 5.8 Anesthetized dog in lateral recumbency for collection of cerebrospinal fluid. (Courtesy of Jodi Carlson, Yale University)

and personal protective equipment should be utilized when collecting and storing radiolabeled samples.

Bone Marrow Collection

Bone marrow is easily collected from dogs at necropsy by opening any of the long bones. If an antemortem sample is needed, **general anesthesia and aseptic technique are usually required.** Local anesthesia will work only with the most cooperative animals. The three most commonly used locations for aspirating bone marrow are the wing of the ilium, the proximal humerus, and the proximal femur. The area over the aspiration site is clipped and aseptically prepped for surgery and sterile surgical gloves are worn. A small stab incision is made through the skin with a scalpel blade and a sterile bone marrow aspiration (Illinois) needle is advanced against the bone at the collection site. The needle is rotated to cut through the cortex into the marrow (Figure 5.9). Once through the cortex, the stylet is removed and the marrow is aspirated. The marrow should be transferred immediately onto microscope slides for evaluation, as it will clot rapidly. If a core sample is needed, a Jamshidi needle is used in place of the Illinois needle. After the cortex is penetrated, the Jamshidi needle is advanced rapidly to cut a cylinder of tissue. The core can be gently rolled along a microscope slide for cytology and then placed in formalin for histopathology.

test article/compound administration techniques

Formulation Guidelines

During drug development and safety testing, nonpharmaceutical-grade formulations are administered to research animals. Commonly, standard vehicles are used to put the test article into solution or suspension for dosing. Because many of these substances are administered parenterally (e.g., intravenously, intramuscularly, intraperitoneally, etc.), institutions should develop procedures to ensure that experimental formulations administered to animals are of an appropriate quality. Factors such as sterility, stability, purity, pyrogenicity, and physicochemical parameters (e.g., pH, osmolality, osmolarity, microbial content) should be considered in order to avoid or minimize adverse effects from the formulation itself. For example, the use of 0.22 μm millipore filters, testing to ensure pyrogen-free status,

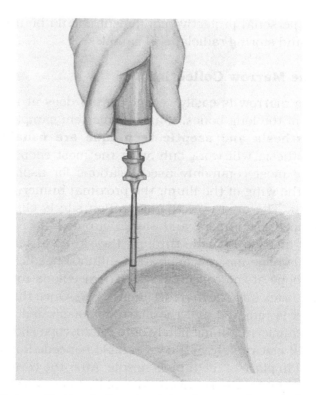

Figure 5.9 Anesthetized dog in lateral recumbency for collection of bone marrow from iliac crest. (Courtesy of Jodi Carlson, Yale University)

and aseptic techniques to prepare formulations will improve sterility and purity. Acceptable ranges of pH and osmolarity should be established. Physiologically normal solutions are preferred, however, acceptable upper and lower limits and criteria for use (e.g., slow infusion or limited volumes for formulations of pH less than 2 or greater than 11) are needed. A compound's solubility and bioavailability may change depending on the vehicle, and by selecting the best formulations, vehicle-specific side effects can be minimized or eliminated.[2,3]

Volume Guidelines

Table 5.1 lists recommended dose volumes for single or multiple dosing and maximum dose volumes appropriate for various routes of administration in the dog. It is recommended that the lowest dose volumes be used whenever possible. Exceeding these limits generally requires scientific justification and IACUC approval. Intramuscular doses should be limited to no more that two per day, as they

TABLE 5.1: RECOMMENDED DOSE VOLUMES

Route	Recommended volumes (single or multiple doses/maximum dose) (ml/kg)
Oral	5/15
Subcutaneous	1/2
Intramuscular	0.25/0.5*
Intraperitoneal	1/20
Intravenous (bolus)	2.5
Intravenous (slow infusion)	5

Per site and maximal total dose.

may be painful, and subcutaneous doses should be limited to two to three sites per day. Bolus intravenous doses are administered within 1 minute or less. Catheters are recommended for slow intravenous infusions, which are typically administered over 5 to 10 minutes, but can take longer depending on solubility or irritancy.[4]

Oral Dosing

When pills are to be administered, they should be appropriately sized for the animal and can be hidden in food treats if doing so will not interfere with the study. Canned dog food, cheese, and peanut butter are useful for hiding pills. If treats cannot be used or if the dog spits out the pill after taking the treat, it may be necessary to administer the pill without food. The dog should be placed in a seated position and the pill should be held between the doser's thumb and index finger. The dog's mouth is gently opened and the pill is pushed back over the tongue as far back into the throat as possible. The dog's mouth is closed and held shut. The ventral neck may be rubbed to induce swallowing. A small amount of water may also be squirted into the dog's mouth to stimulate swallowing.

When liquids must be administered, they can be placed in a gelatin capsule for dosing. If gavage is needed, a mouth gag is placed to prevent the dog from biting down on the tube. If a gag is unavailable, a roll of bandage tape can be used as a temporary substitute. The tube (3 to 5 French) is placed through the gag, over the tongue, and down the throat. The length of the tube needed to reach the stomach is approximately three-fourths of the distance from the tip of the nose to the last rib. If the tube is located correctly, it can be palpated in the throat just behind the trachea. If the tube has been inadvertently placed in the trachea, only the trachea can be palpated, and the dog may cough or gag. Liquids should never be infused into a gavage tube unless placement in the stomach can be confirmed. Unintentional infusion of liquids into the lungs can cause immediate death or, if the animal survives, severe pneumonia.

Nasogastric tube administration can be used as a substitute for orogastric administration. For nasogastric administration, a small-diameter flexible tube is lubricated with a water-soluble lubricant and passed into a nostril to the back of the throat until swallowed. Once swallowed, the tube is passed into the stomach, as for an oro-gastric tube.[4]

Injection Sites

Intravenous injections can be made into the cephalic, saphenous, or jugular veins. The needle is inserted into the vein as for drawing blood, a small volume of blood is aspirated back to ensure the needle is in the vein, and the injection is made. If multiple injections are to be made over a short period of time, an indwelling catheter may be placed. The use of a catheter is also preferred if the solution might cause irritation if extravascular leakage occurs. After injecting the material into the catheter, 1 to 3 ml of saline should be injected to prevent some of the solution from remaining in the catheter. If multiple injections are to be placed over a long period of time, use of a vascular access port may be preferred.

Intramuscular injections are most often made in the biceps femoris muscle just caudal to the femur. The next most commonly used muscles are the paravertebral muscles parallel to the spine. The quadriceps muscles just cranial to the femur and the triceps muscle just caudal to the humerus are also occasionally used. Caution must be used to avoid injecting around nerves or into a blood vessel. The absence of a "flash" of blood in the syringe when drawing back on it before injecting will help prevent injections into a vein or artery.

Subcutaneous injections may be made anywhere along the trunk, but the most common location is under the loose skin between the shoulder blades.

Implantable Osmotic Minipumps

For continuous infusions of small volumes of liquid, osmotic mini-pumps are ideal. The compound to be administered is loaded into the pump, and the pump is placed into the location where the fluid should be delivered, usually subcutaneously or intraperitoneally. If intravenous infusion is desired, the pump can be attached to a sur-

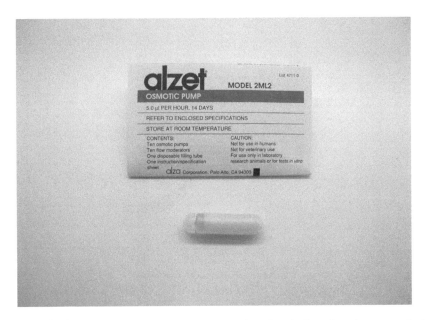

Figure 5.10 Osmotic minipumps are implanted subcutaneously in the dorsal neck/upper back area for controlled delivery of test articles over longer periods of time.

gically implanted intravenous cannula. Minipumps operate by diffusion of water through a semipermeable membrane into the pump housing. The diffusion of water into the pump forces out the compound at a slow, but continuous rate. Depending on the size and type of pump used, solution can be continuously administered for up to 4 weeks (Figure 5.10). Protective jackets or collars may be required to prevent dogs from disturbing the implantation site (Figure 5.11 and Figure 5.12).

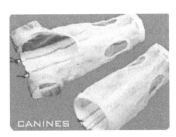

Figure 5.11 Dog jackets are used to protect surgical sites or hold data collection equipment, such as a Holter monitor for continuous recording of the heart's rhythm. (Courtesy of Teresa Price, Lomir Biomedical)

telemetry

A wide variety of implantable telemetry devices are available for dogs. These devices allow the collection of physiologic data at baseline levels while the animal is at rest in its home cage. Most laboratory dogs rest quietly in

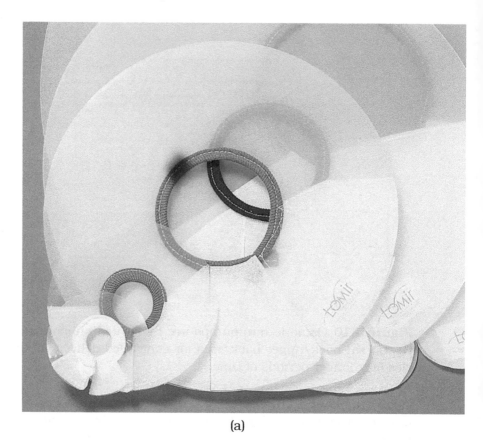

(a)

Figure 5.12 Protective collars include (a) traditional Elizabethan, (b) cervical, which doesn't impair vision, and (c) a padded pillow collar. (Courtesy of Teresa Price, Lomir Biomedical)

their cages except when a caretaker or an investigator enters the room. The presence of the caretaker or investigator causes excitement and, therefore, increases heart rate, blood pressure, etc. As the dogs become accustomed to the presence of the individual, the excitement diminishes, and the physiologic parameters return to their baseline values. Sudden movements or noises caused by the individual can cause additional excitement and another change in the physiologic parameters.

The use of telemetry allows data to be collected without the investigator being present in the room. Depending on the type of data to be collected, one or more telemetry devices are aseptically implanted into the dog by an experienced surgeon. Implants (Figure 5.13) are available for measuring blood pressure, heart rate, body tempera-

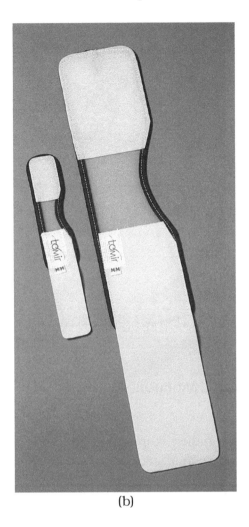

(b)

Figure 5.12 (continued)

ture, electrocardiograms (ECGs or EKGs: electrical activity of the heart), electroencephalograms (EEGs: electrical activity of the brain), and even electromyograms (EMGs: electrical activity of muscles). The implants take measurements and transmit the data to a receiver kept near the animal's cage. The receiver is normally connected to a computer that stores the data and allows it to be evaluated at the investigator's convenience. Many of the implants can be turned on and off using a remote control to save battery life when data is not being collected. By evaluating data collected while the animal is in a true resting state, not excited from the presence of an investigator or

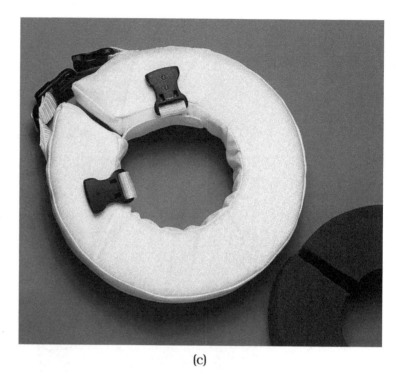

(c)

Figure 5.12 (continued)

caretaker, smaller, more subtle differences caused by experimental drugs or other treatments can be detected.

---

necropsy

For research purposes, necropsy generally involves removal and collection of one or more organs important to the research project. For general toxicology studies, however, all organs are examined in a systematic fashion. Diagnostic necropsies vary in complexity, but records of such should be maintained as part of the animal's permanent medical record (also discussed in Chapter 2).

The first step in a necropsy is euthanasia. Recommendations for euthanasia methods have been published by the American Veterinary Medical Association Panel on Euthanasia.[5] Overdose of a barbiturate-containing euthanasia solution is the most commonly used method. For toxicology studies where excellent histopathology is essential, exsanguination under euthanasia is the preferred method.

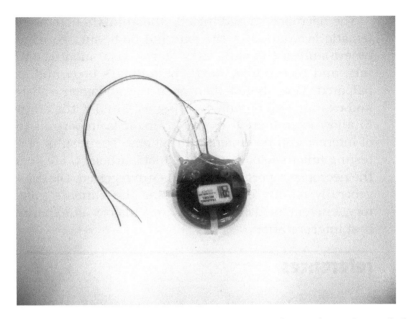

Figure 5.13 Telemetry device used for recording physiological data such as EKG, EEG blood pressure and temperature.

Exsanguination rids the tissues of excess blood and improves the veterinary pathologists' ability to see minor changes in tissues.

Ideally the necropsy should be performed immediately after death to avoid postmortem autolysis. If the animal cannot be necropsied immediately, it should be refrigerated. Freezing must be avoided if histopathology is planned, as freezing damages the cellular architecture. Necropsies should be performed in a well-lit necropsy room, preferably on a downdraft table.

Basic instruments include a large scale to obtain the dog's body weight and a smaller scale to weigh organs. A scalpel, sharp scissors, forceps, and bone cutting tools are also needed. Containers filled with 10% neutral buffered formalin solution are used to store tissues or organs saved for further evaluation. As a general rule, in order to ensure proper tissue fixation, one should use a 10:1 to 20:1 ratio of formalin to tissues and tissues should be cut into slices no more than about 0.5 cm thick. Specimen sampling containers and devices (sterile swabs and culturettes, syringe-needle sets and specimen vials, etc.) or imaging studies (radiographs, magnetic resonance imaging, computed tomography, etc.) may also be needed, depending on the type of necropsy.

The necropsy should include the animal's body weight and a systematic evaluation of the external body surface. One should start by evaluating the skin, eyes, ears, nose, mouth, oral cavity, genitals, and rectal area. Next, the animal's body and extremities are palpated. One should then open the abdomen and thoracic cavity and examine all organs and tissues. Finally, the cranium is opened to allow examination of the brain. It is important to save tissues of interest and document all findings. The results of any additional testing (microbiology, imaging, histopathology, etc.) can be added to the necropsy report when results are received. Diagnostic necropsies generally require details regarding the animal's past medical history, current medical history, and history of experimental use for best interpretation.

references

1. Removal of blood from laboratory mammals and birds, First report of the BVA/FRAME/RSPCA/UFAW Joint Working Group on Refinement, *Lab. Anim.*, 17, 1, 1993.

2. Wolf, A., Garnett, N., Potkay, S., Wigglesworth, C., Doyle, D., and Thornton, V., Frequently asked questions about the Public Health Service policy on humane care and use of laboratory animals, *Lab. Animal*, 32(9), 33, 2003.

3. Morton, D.B., Jennings, M., Buckwell, A., Ewbank, R., Godfrey, C., Holgate, B., Inglis, I., James, R., Page, C., Sharman, I., Verschoyle, R., Westall, L., Wilson, A.B., and Joint Working Group on Refinement, Refining procedures for the administration of substances, Report of the BVAAWF/FRAME/RSPCA/UFAW Joint Working Group on Refinement, British Veterinary Association Animal Welfare Foundation/Fund for the Replacement of Animals in Medical Experiments/Royal Society for the Prevention of Cruelty to Animals/Universities Federation for Animal Welfare, *Lab. Anim.*, 35, 1, 2001.

4. Diehl, K.L., Hull, D., Morton, D., Phister, R., Rabemampianina, Y., Smith, D., Vidal, J.-M., and Vorstenbosch, C.V.D., A good practice guide to the administration of- substances and removal of blood, including routes and volumes, *J. Appl. Toxicol.*, 21, 15, 2001.

5. AVMA Panel on Euthanasia, American Veterinary Medical Association, 2000 Report of the AVMA Panel on Euthanasia, *J. Am. Vet. Med. Assoc.*, 218, 669, 2001.

resources

This chapter provides selected information on relevant organizations and vendors as sources of information regarding dogs, laboratory equipment, and materials and resources such as journals, books, electronic databases, etc., important to laboratory animal users. The lists are not exhaustive, nor do they imply endorsement of one vendor over another; rather, they are provided to serve as a starting point for developing a database of resources.

organizations

Numerous professional affiliated organizations exist that can provide initial contacts for obtaining information regarding specific professional issues related to the care and use of laboratory canines. One should consider individual or institutional membership in these organizations as a means of acquiring knowledge on current regulatory issues, veterinary care and animal health issues, new techniques and equipment, emerging diseases, management issues, publications, meetings, and other related issues. Relevant organizations include the following:

American Association for Laboratory Animal Science (AALAS), 9190 Crestwyn Hills Drive, Memphis, TN 38125-8538 (Telephone: 901-754-8620; Fax: 901-753-0046; e-mail: info@aalas. org; website: http://www.aalas.org/). AALAS is a cornerstone organization for the laboratory animal community, dedicated to the advancement of the responsible care and use of laboratory animals in the conduct of quality science for the benefit of human and animal health and the advancement of science. AALAS serves the needs of a diverse constituency, including animal caretakers, technicians, researchers, veterinarians, Institutional Animal Care and Use Committee (IACUC) members, animal breeders, and equipment and supply vendors, among others. Through publication of the journals *Comparative Medicine* and the *Journal of the American Association for Laboratory Animal Science* (JAALAS; formerly called *Contemporary Topics in Laboratory Animal Science*) and the bimonthly newsletter *TechTalk*, it provides ongoing education and communication to its members. Through its sponsorship of programs to certify laboratory animal professionals as Assistant Laboratory Animal Technician (ALAT), Laboratory Animal Technician (LAT), Laboratory Animal Technologist (LATG), and Certified Manager of Animal Resources (CMAR), it provides enhanced professionalism and ongoing training to its members. Through the affiliated Institute for Laboratory Animal Management (ILAM) program it provides advanced training in laboratory animal facility management to members. AALAS maintains a resource-laden website that includes extensive links to relevant organizations, regulatory agencies, and resource materials related to laboratory animal management. AALAS also sponsors or hosts forums for ongoing member communications, such as TechLink and COMPMED (Comparative Medicine Discussion List). AALAS sponsors an annual meeting and has numerous local branch affiliations.

American College of Laboratory Animal Medicine (ACLAM), contact information is available at their website: http://www.aclam. org/. ACLAM is an organization of laboratory animal veterinarians founded to encourage education, training, and research in laboratory animal medicine. ACLAM is dedicated to humane, proper, and safe care and use of laboratory animals. ACLAM is recognized as a specialty of veterinary medicine by the American Veterinary Medical Association (AVMA) and establishes standards of education, training, experience, and expertise necessary to become qualified as a specialist, culminating in certification as a diplomate through passing a certifying exam. ACLAM promotes the advancement of knowledge in this field through sponsorship of an annual forum, commonly dedicated to a particular topic of interest, sessions at the AVMA and AALAS meetings, publication of a quarterly newsletter and texts such as *Laboratory Animal Medicine* (Academic Press, San Diego), the development of a series of autotutorials on laboratory animals, and other means. ACLAM fosters the recognition of its members who contribute to improving human and animal health by being the leaders of the veterinary medical specialty known as laboratory animal medicine.

American Society of Laboratory Animal Practitioners (ASLAP), ASLAP Coordinator, P.O. Box 125, Adamstown, MD 21710

(Telephone: 301-874-4826; Fax: 301-874-6195; e-mail: aslap-info@ aslap.org; website: http://www.aslap.org/). ASLAP is an organization of veterinarians and veterinary students practicing or having an interest in laboratory animal medicine. ASLAP's mission is to promote the acquisition and dissemination of knowledge, ideas, and information for the benefit of laboratory animals, other animals, and society in general, and as an organization it strives to define, meet, and improve upon the veterinary needs of laboratory animals. ASLAP promotes education, training, and communication through publication of a newsletter and sponsorship of annual meetings in conjunction with AALAS or AVMA meetings.

American Veterinary Medical Association (AVMA), 1931 North Meacham Road, Suite 100, Schaumburg, IL 60173 (Telephone: 847-925-8070; Fax: 847-925-1329; e-mail: avmainfo@avma.org; website: http://www.avma.org/). The AVMA is the cornerstone organization of veterinarians in the United States working in all areas of veterinary medicine, including laboratory animal medicine. The AVMA's mission is to improve animal and human health and advance the profession of veterinary medicine. The AVMA promotes communication, training, and the advancement of knowledge in veterinary medicine through its journal publications, such as the *Journal of the American Veterinary Medical Association* and the *American Journal of Veterinary Research*, sponsorship of the Network of Animal Health (NOAH) forum and annual meetings, and other informational resources on their website.

Animal Welfare Information Center (AWIC), U.S. Department of Agriculture, Agricultural Research Service, National Agricultural Library, 10301 Baltimore Avenue, 4th Floor, Beltsville, MD 20705-2351 (Telephone: 301-504-6212; Fax: 301-504-7125; e-mail: awic@ nal.usda.gov; website: http://www.nal.usda.gov/awic/). The AWIC is part of the U.S. Department of Agriculture (USDA) library (National Agricultural Library) and was founded under the provisions of an amendment to the Animal Welfare Act to serve as an informational resource. Through its website, the AWIC provides a wide variety of informational resources to the research community, including proper care and use of laboratory animals, alternatives to animal testing in research and education, training materials for laboratory animal personnel and investigators using animals, improved and refined research methodologies, animal care and use committees, and other related areas. The AWIC sponsors workshops and provides onsite training to assist institutions in understanding and meeting the informational requirements of the animal welfare regulations, including training information specialists on how to conduct comprehensive alternatives searches.

Association for Assessment and Accreditation of Laboratory Animal Care, International (AAALAC), 5283 Corporate Drive, Suite 203, Frederick, MD 21703 (Telephone: 301-696-9626; Fax: 301-696-9627; e-mail: accredit@aaalac.org; website: http://www.aaalac.org/). The AAALAC is a nonprofit organization that promotes the humane care and use of animals through provision of an independent mechanism for peer evaluation of animal care programs. The AAALAC accreditation process is voluntary and includes a comprehensive program review using the *Guide for the Care and Use of Laboratory Animals* as a guideline. Achieving AAALAC accreditation has been widely accepted as strong evidence (a "gold standard") of an institution having a high-quality animal care program. Institutions achieving accreditation represent the broad spectrum of animal research facilities, including medical schools, universities, governmental agencies, animal breeders, and biotechnology and pharmaceutical companies.

Canadian Council on Animal Care (CCAC), 130 Albert Street, Suite 1510, Ottawa, ON, Canada K1P 5G4 (Telephone: 613-238-4031, ext. 32; Fax: 613-238-2837; e-mail: ccac@ccac.ca; website: www.ccac.ca). The CCAC is a nonprofit, national peer review agency in Canada whose mission is to set and maintain standards for the care and use of animals used in research, teaching, and testing. Membership includes governmental agencies, universities, pharmaceutical companies, the Canadian Association for Laboratory Animal Science (CALAS), and medical research societies. CCAC conducts assessments of animal care programs using the CCAC *Guide to the Care and Use of Experimental Animals* as guidelines.

Center for Alternatives to Animal Testing (CAAT), 615 N. Wolfe Street, Baltimore, MD 21205 (Telephone: 443-287-7277; e-mail: caat@jhsph.edu; website: http://caat.jhsph.edu/). The CAAT is an academic center affiliated with the Division of Toxicological Sciences in the Department of Environmental Health Sciences of the Johns Hopkins University Bloomberg School of Public Health. CAAT's mission is to be a leading force in the development and use of reduction, refinement, and replacement alternatives in research, testing, and education to protect and enhance the health of the public. Through the provision of funding for alternatives research, sponsorship of meetings, and *Altweb* (Alternatives to Animal Testing on the Web), CAAT promotes communication, education, training, and the advancement of knowledge in alternatives to the use of animals in research.

Federation of European Laboratory Animal Science Associations (FELASA), 25 Shaftesbury Avenue, London W1D 7EG, United Kingdom (e-mail: jguillen@unav.es; website: http://www.felasa.org). FELASA is a nonprofit organization composed of various European national and local laboratory animal associations dedicated to education and training for those engaged in the provision of care or use of laboratory animals and animal health monitoring. FELASA promotes advancement of knowledge in this field through sponsorship of triennial international conferences, sponsorship of programs to accredit teaching programs for training laboratory animal technicians, research technicians, scientists, and specialists, and sponsorship of working groups such as the ECLAM/ESLAV/FELASA Working Group on Veterinary Care.

Foundation for Biomedical Research (FBR), 818 Connecticut Avenue NW, Suite 900, Washington, DC 20006 (Telephone: 202-457-0654; Fax: 202-457-0659; e-mail: info@fbresearch.org; website: http://www.fbresearch.org/). The FBR is a nonprofit organization dedicated to improving human and animal health by promoting public understanding and support for the humane and responsible use of animals in medical and scientific research. Through sponsorship of educational programs, informational resources, and the Michael E. DeBakey Journalism Awards, FBR provides a voice for the advancement of science through the use of animals in research. FBR is a sister organization to the National Association for Biomedical Research (NABR).

Institute of Laboratory Animal Research (ILAR), The Keck Center of the National Academy of Sciences, 500 Fifth Street NW, Washington, DC 20001 (Telephone: 202-334-2590; Fax: 202-334-1687; e-mail: ILAR@nas.edu; website: http://dels.nas.edu/ilar_n/ilarhome/). ILAR is an agency within the National Academy of Sciences that acts in an advisory capacity to the federal government, the biomedical research community, and the public. ILAR develops guidelines and provides information on the care and use of animals in research. ILAR publishes reports, books, and journals such as the *ILAR Journal* as an informational resource to the research community.

International Council for Laboratory Animal Science (ICLAS) (website: http://www.iclas.org/). ICLAS is an international, nonprofit scientific organization dedicated to advancing human and animal health by promoting the ethical care and use of laboratory animals in research worldwide. ICLAS promotes international collaboration in laboratory animal science, worldwide harmonization in the care and use of laboratory animals, and dissemination of information on laboratory animal science.

Laboratory Animal Management Association (LAMA) (website: http://www.lama-online.org/). LAMA is a nonprofit organization dedicated to enhancing the quality of management and care of laboratory animals throughout the world. LAMA promotes professional education and training through sponsorship of seminars, workshops, and an annual meeting, normally held in conjunction with the annual AALAS meeting and publication of *LAMA Lines* and *LAMA Review.*

National Association for Biomedical Research (NABR), 818 Connecticut Avenue NW, Suite 900, Washington, DC 20006 (Telephone: 202-857-0540; Fax: 202-659-1902; e-mail: info@nabr.org; website: http://www.nabr.org/). NABR is a nonprofit organization dedicated solely to advocating sound public policy that recognizes the vital role of humane animal use in biomedical research, higher education, and product safety testing. NABR provides a voice for the research community regarding legislative and regulatory matters affecting laboratory animal research. NABR is a sister organization to the Foundation for Biomedical Research (FBR).

Office of Laboratory Animal Welfare (OLAW), National Institutes of Health, RKL1, Suite 360, MSC 7982, 6705 Rockledge Drive, Bethesda, MD 20892-7982 (Telephone: 301-496-7163; Fax: 301-402-2803; e-mail: olaw@od.nih.gov; website: http://grants.nih.gov/grants/olaw/olaw.htm). OLAW is an agency within the Office of Extramural Research (OER) of the National Institutes of Health (NIH) charged with the development of appropriate policies and procedures and compliance oversight relative to the Public Health Service Policy on Humane Care and Use of Laboratory Animals. This policy concerns research conducted or supported by any component of the Public Health Service.

Public Responsibility in Medicine and Research (PRIM&R), 126 Brookline Avenue, Suite 202, Boston, MA 02215-3920 (Telephone: 617-423-4112; Fax: 617-423-1185; e-mail: info@primr.org; website: http://www.primr.org/). PRIM&R is a nonprofit organization serving a diverse constituency, including animal caretakers, researchers, veterinarians, and administrators from academia, the pharmaceutical industry, and the government involved in the care and use of animals. PRIM&R is dedicated to creating, implementing, and advancing the highest ethical standards in the conduct of research and through sponsorship of meetings, educational programs, and training resources serves the biomedical research community. PRIM&R is sister organization to Applied Research Ethics National Association (ARENA).

Scientists Center for Animal Welfare (SCAW), 7833 Walker Drive, Suite 410, Greenbelt, MD 20770 (Telephone: 301-345-3500; Fax: 301-345-3503; e-mail: info@scaw.com; website: http://www.scaw.com). SCAW is a nonprofit educational association of individuals and institutions whose mission is to promote humane care, use, and management of animals involved in research, testing, and education in laboratory, agriculture, wildlife, or other settings. SCAW promotes the advancement of knowledge in this field through sponsorship of conferences, workshops, forums for ongoing member communications such as *IACUC Talk*, and various publications including the quarterly *SCAW Newsletter*.

Society of Toxicology (SOT), 1821 Michael Faraday Drive, Suite 300, Reston VA 20190 (Telephone: 703-438-3115; Fax: 703-438-3113; e-mail: sothq@toxicology.org; website: http://www.toxicology.org/). The SOT is a nonprofit organization comprised of scientists from academia, the pharmaceutical industry, and the government involved in toxicology, whose mission is to advance science to enhance human, animal, and environmental health. SOT promotes the advancement of knowledge in this field through sponsorship of conferences, workshops, continuing education, educational outreach programs, and various publications such as the journal *Toxicological Sciences*. SOT has numerous local branch affiliations that sponsor meetings throughout the year.

U.S. Department of Agriculture, Animal and Plant Health Inspection Service, Animal Care (USDA, APHIS, AC), 4700 River Road, Unit 84, Riverdale, MD 20737-1234 (Telephone: 301-734-7833; Fax: 301-734-4978; e-mail: ace@aphis.usda.gov; website: http://www.aphis.usda.gov/ac/). Animal Care is an agency within APHIS, which is part of the USDA and is responsible for administering the Animal Welfare Act. Through development of acceptable standards of humane animal care and treatment and using compliance inspections, AC ensures that minimum standards of care and treatment are provided for dogs used in research or exhibited to the public. Other warm-blooded mammals exhibited in zoos, circuses, and marine mammal facilities and pets transported on commercial airlines are also regulated by APHIS.

U.S. Food and Drug Administration (FDA), 5600 Fishers Lane, Rockville, MD 20857-0001 (Telephone: 1-888-INFO-FDA/1-888-463-6332; e-mail contact through website: http://www.fda.gov/comments.html; website: http://www.fda.gov/). The FDA is an agency within the

U.S. Department of Health and Human Services. The FDA is responsible for protecting the public health by ensuring the safety, efficacy, and security of human and veterinary drugs, biological products, medical devices, the U.S. food supply, cosmetics, and products that emit radiation. Under mandate of the Federal Food and Drug Act of 1906 and as amended, the FDA has oversight of preclinical safety testing of drugs in animals. FDA promulgated the good laboratory practices (GLPs) as standards to guide such testing. The National Center for Toxicological Research (NCTR) is an agency within the FDA that performs consumer product safety/toxicity testing in animals.

publications

Representative publications, including books and periodicals of interest to laboratory animal professionals are listed below.

Books

1. *Anesthesia and Analgesia in Laboratory Animals.* Kohn, D.G., Wixson, S.K., White, W.J., and Benson, J.G., eds., 1997. Academic Press, New York, NY 10010 (Telephone: 800-321-5068; website: www.academicpress.com).

2. *The ARENA/OLAW Institutional Animal Care and Use Committee Guidebook,* 2nd ed. Pitts, M., Bayne, K., Anderson, L.C., Benhardt, D.B., Greene, M., Klemfuss, H., Oki, G.S.F., Rozmiarek, H., Theran, P., and Van Sluyters, P.C., eds., 2002. OLAW, NIH, Bethesda, MD 20892-7982. The book is available as a free downloadable PDF file online at http://grants.nih.gov/grants/olaw/olaw.htm.

3. *Biosafety in Microbiological and Biomedical Laboratories,* 4th ed. CDC-NIH (Centers for Disease Control and Prevention–National Institutes of Health), 1999. HHS Publication no. (CDC) 93-8395, U.S. Government Printing Office, Washington, DC 20402 (Telephone: 202-257-3318). This book can be read free online at http://bmbl.od.nih.gov/.

4. *Formulary for Laboratory Animals,* 2nd ed. Hawk, C.T. and Leary, S.L., eds., 1999. Iowa State University Press, Ames, IA 50014 (Telephone: 800-862-6657; website: http://www.isu-press.edu).

5. *Guide for the Care and Use of Laboratory Animals,* 7th ed. National Research Council, Institute for Laboratory Animal

Resources Committee to Revise the Guide for the Care and Use of Laboratory Animals, 1996. National Academy Press, Washington, DC (Telephone: 888-624-8373; website: htpp://www.nap.edu).

6. *Laboratory Animal Anesthesia*, 2nd ed. Flecknell, P.A., 1996. Academic Press, San Diego, CA 92101-4495 (Telephone: 800-321-5068; website: www.academicpress.com).

7. *Laboratory Animal Medicine*, 2nd ed. Fox, J.G., Anderson. L.C., Loew, F.M., and Quimby, F.W., eds., 2002. Academic Press, San Diego, CA 92101-4495 (Telephone: 800-321-5068; website: www.academicpress.com).

8. *Management of Laboratory Animal Care and Use Programs*. Suckow, M.A., Douglas, F.A., and Weichbrod, R.H., eds., 2002. CRC Press, Boca Raton, FL 33431 (Telephone: 800-272-7737; website: http://www.crcpress.com/).

Periodicals

1. *American Journal of Veterinary Research*, published by the American Veterinary Medical Association; website: http://www.avma.org/.

2. *Comparative Medicine*, published by American Association for Laboratory Animal Science. Available online at http://www.aalas.org/.

3. *ILAR Journal*, published by the Institute of Laboratory Animal Research, National Research Council. Older articles are available free online and current articles are available free to members at http://dels.nas.edu/ilar_n/ilarhome/.

4. *Journal of the American Association for Laboratory Animal Science* (formerly *Contemporary Topics in Laboratory Animal Science*), published by the American Association for Laboratory Animal Science. Available online at http://www.aalas.org/.

5. *Journal of the American Veterinary Medical Association*, published by the American Veterinary Medical Association; website: http://www.avma.org/.

6. *Lab Animal*, published by Nature Publishing Co., New York, NY 10010-1707. Articles are available free online at http://www.nature.com/laban/index.html.

7.   *Laboratory Animals*, published by the Royal Society of Medicine Press, London, WIG OAE, United Kingdom; website: http://www.lal.org.uk/.

electronic resources

Many online sources of information relevant to the care and use of laboratory animals, including canines, are available. These include the following:

1.   **American Association for Laboratory Animal Science (AALAS).** AALAS maintains a resource-laden website at http://www.aalas.org/ that includes extensive links to relevant organizations, regulatory agencies, and resource materials related to laboratory animal management. AALAS sponsors or hosts forums for ongoing member communications, such as TechLink, COMPMED (Comparative Medicine Discussion List), and IACUC Forum. COMPMED is an electronic mailing list available to laboratory animal science professionals worldwide, including animal caretakers, veterinarians, researchers, and administrators. It serves as a forum for the exchange of information on all species of laboratory animals and related topics in biomedical research with professionals in the field of laboratory animal science. Members can submit questions and it has a searchable archives. The AALAS Learning Library offers free and paid courses for members at individual and group rates. Courses offered cover topics such as regulations, methods, and the care, handling, and use of laboratory animals. Courses are helpful when preparing for AALAS certification exams or obtaining continuing education credits.

2.   **Animal Welfare Information Center (AWIC).** The AWIC website at http://www.nal.usda.gov/awic/ provides numerous informational resources to the research community on subjects related to the proper care and use of laboratory animals and alternatives to animal testing in research and education. It contains searchable databases, reference databases, training materials, and other relevant resources.

3.   **Comparative Medicine Discussion List (COMPMED).** COMPMED is an AALAS-sponsored electronic mailing list available to laboratory animal science professionals worldwide including animal caretakers, veterinarians, researchers

and administrators. Its purpose is to serve as a forum for the exchange of information on all species of laboratory animals and related topics in biomedical research with professionals in the field of laboratory animal science. Members can submit questions to the list and COMPMED has searchable archives to look for answers to previously asked questions.

4. **International Veterinary Information Service (IVIS).** IVIS is a nonprofit organization whose goal is to provide information to veterinarians, veterinary students, and animal health professionals. Its website provides access to electronic books, proceedings of veterinary meetings, short courses, continuing education (lecture notes, manuals, auto tutorials, and interactive websites), an international meeting calendar, image collections, links to other sites, and other items of interest to laboratory animal professionals. Additional information is available by contacting IVIS at P.O. Box 4371, Ithaca, NY 14852 (e-mail: info@ivis.org; website: http://www.ivis.org/).

5. **NetVet Veterinary Resources and Electronic Zoo (NetVet).** This website contains a comprehensive listing of directories and links on veterinary medicine and veterinary resources of interest to laboratory animal professionals, including mailing lists, newsgroups, publications, regulations, policies, animals, etc. It was developed by Dr. Ken Boschert of Washington University, St. Louis, Missouri, and is licensed by the AVMA. For more information, visit the website: http://netvet. wustl.edu/e-zoo.

6. **Network of Animal Health (NOAH).** NOAH is an online service sponsored by the AVMA and available to AVMA members. It offers a forum for exchange of information, links to various databases, drug references to veterinary pharmaceuticals and biologicals, and other resources of interest to laboratory animal professionals. Additional information is available from the American Veterinary Medical Association, 1931 North Meacham Road, Suite 100, Schaumburg, IL 60173 (Telephone: 847-925-8070; Fax: 847-925-1329; e-mail: avmainfo@avma.org; website: http://www.avma.org/).

canine sources

Various breeds of purpose-bred dogs (beagles, mongrels, etc.) may be acquired through vendors. Random-source dogs of various breeds may be acquired through USDA class B dealers or local shelters or pounds (where allowed). Representative sources for purchasing dogs are listed, but one should consult the *Lab Animal* buyers guide for additional sources of dogs. When acquiring dogs, it is important to obtain animals that meet internal health standards and requirements. Ensuring that your vendor has a proper conditioning program for dogs, including veterinary checks, vaccinations, anthelmintics, socialization, etc., is important. Examples of purpose-bred dog vendors include the following:

1. Barton's West End Facilities, 161 Janes Chapel Road, Oxford, NJ 07863 (Telephone: 908-637-4427; e-mail: bwef@bwefinc.com).

2. Covance Research Products, P.O. Box 7200, Denver, PA 17517 (Telephone: 717-336-4921; e-mail: info@crpinc.com; website: http://www.crpinc.com).

3. Harlan, P.O. Box 29176, Indianapolis, IN 46229 (Telephone: 317-894-7521; e-mail: harlan@harlan.com; website: http://www.harlan.com).

4. Haycock Kennels, 629 Apple Road, Quakertown, PA 18951 (Telephone: 215-536-8228).

5. Marshall BioResources (Farms), 5800 Lake Bluff Road, North Rose, NY 14516 (Telephone: 315-587-2295; e-mail: info@marshallbio.com).

6. Ridglan Farms, P.O. Box 318, Mt. Horeb, WI 53572 (Telephone: 608-437-8670; e-mail: ridglan@mhtc.net).

transportation services/resources

Listed below are some organizations that can provide helpful information or services regarding the transportation of dogs. In addition, most canine vendors/breeders offer delivery of animals to the purchasing facility.

1. Animal Transportation Association (AATA), 111 East Loop North, Houston, TX 77029 (Telephone: 713-532-2177; Fax: 713-532-2166; e-mail: info@aata-animaltransport.org; website: http://www.aata-animaltransport.org).

2. Frame's Animal Transportation Service/Custom Crating, 1119 Haverford Road, Ridley Park, PA 19078 (Telephone: 610-521-1123; Fax: 610-521-5651).

3. International Air Transport Association (IATA), 800 Place Victoria, P.O. Box 113, Montreal, Quebec, Canada H4Z 1M1 (Telephone: +1 514-874-0202; e-mail: custserv@iata.org; website: http://www.iata.org/index).

laboratory services

Listed below are some commercial laboratories that provide diagnostic testing services, such as clinical pathology and histopathology for canines.

1. Antech Diagnostics. 1111 Marcus Avenue, Suite M2B, Lake Success, NY 11042 (Telephone: 800-872-1001; website: http://www.antechdiagnostics.com).

2. Bio Reliance. 14920 Broschart Road, Rockville, MD 20850 (Telephone: 800-553-5372; Fax: 301-610-9087; e-mail: info@ bioreliance.com; website: http://www.bioreliance.com).

feed

A variety of diets are available for general use. Representative sources for standard diets, certified diets, and specialty diets are listed. Standards applied to diet vendors should also extend to local distributors of diets. Specialty diets encompass a wide variety of diets, including reformulations of standard diets with variable fat content or mixed with test compounds or medications.

1. Bio-Serv, 1 8th St., Frenchtown, NJ 08825 (Telephone: 908-996-2155 or 800-996-9908; Fax: 908-996-4123; e-mail: sales@bio-serv.com; website: http://www.bio-serv.com).

2. Harlan Teklad, P.O. Box 44220, Madison, WI 53744 (Telephone: 608-277-2070 or 800-4-TEKLAD; Fax: 608-277-2066; e-mail: teklad@teklad.com; website: http://www.teklad.com).

3. 63141 (Telephone: 314-317-5180 or 800-227-8941; Fax: 314-317-5276; website: http://www.labdiet.com).

4. Research Diets, Inc., 20 Jules Lane, New Brunswick, NJ 08901 (Telephone: 732-247-2390 or 877-486-2486; Fax: 732-247-2340; e-mail: info@researchdiets.com; website: http://www.researchdiets.com).

5. Zeigler Brothers, P.O. Box 95, Gardners, PA 17324 (Telephone: 717-677-6181 or 800-841-6800; Fax: 717-677-6826; e-mail: sales@zeiglerfeed.com; website: http://www.zeiglerfeed.com).

equipment

Sanitation

Sources of sanitation chemicals, equipment, and supplies are listed below. See the *Lab Animal* buyers guide for additional sources.

1. BioSentry, 1481 Rock Mountain Boulevard, Stone Mountain, GA 30083 (Telephone: 770-723-9211 or 800-788-4246; Fax: 770-723-7056; e-mail: info@biosentry.com; website: http://www.biosentry.com).

2. Charm Sciences Inc., 659 Andover Street, Lawrence, MA 01843 (Telephone: 978-687-9200; e-mail: customerservice@ charm.com; website: http://www.charm.com).

3. Getinge USA, Inc. 1777 East Henrietta Road, Rochester, NY 14623 (Telephone: 585-475-1400 or 800-475-9040; Fax: 585-272-5116; e-mail: info@getingeusa.com; website: http://www. getingeusa.com).

4. Girton Manufacturing Company, Inc., 160 W. Main Street, Millville, PA 17846 (Telephone: 570-458-5521; Fax: 570-458-5589; website: http://www.girton.com).

5. Pharmacal Research Labs, P.O. Box 369, Naugatuck, CT 06770 (Telephone: 203-755-4908 or 800-243-5350; Fax: 203-755-4309; e-mail: moreinfo@pharmacal.com; website: http:// www.pharmacal.com).

6. Quip Laboratories, Inc., 1500 Eastlawn Avenue, Wilmington, DE 19802 (Telephone: 302-761-2600 or 800-424-2436; Fax: 302-761-2611; website: http://www.quiplabs.com).

7. Rochester Midland Corp., 333 Hollenbeck Street, Rochester, NY 14621 (Telephone: 585-336-2376 or 800-836-1627; Fax: 716-336-2357; website: http://www.rochestermidland.com).

8. Scientek Hospital & Laboratory Equipment, 11151 Bridgeport Road, Richmond, British Columbia, Canada V6X 1T3 (Telephone: 604-273-9094 or 866-321-3828; Fax: 604-273-1262; e-mail: sales@scientek.net; website: http://www.scientek.net).

9. Steris Corporation, 5960 Heisley Road, Mentor, OH 44060 (Telephone: 440-354-2600 or 800-444-9009; Fax: 440-357-2321; website: http://www.steris.com).

Cages, Research, and Veterinary Supplies

Multiple sources for pharmaceuticals, hypodermic needles, syringes, surgical equipment, bandages, and other related items are listed below. Pharmaceuticals should be ordered and used only under the direction of a veterinarian. Cages should meet the size requirements as specified by relevant regulatory agencies. Stainless steel is preferable to galvanized steel.

TABLE 6.1: POSSIBLE COMMERCIAL SOURCES OF CAGES AND RESEARCH AND VETERINARY SUPPLIES

Item	Sources
Cages and supplies	2, 3, 5, 8, 15–18, 21, 23
Veterinary and surgical supplies	9–11, 13, 20, 26
Gas anesthesia equipment	11, 20, 22
Handling and restraint equipment	19
Enrichment devices/treats	6
Syringes and needles	11, 12, 20, 24–26
Vascular access equipment	1, 7, 14
Osmotic pumps	4
Necropsy tools	12

1. Access Technologies, 7350 N. Ridgeway, Skokie, IL 60076 (Telephone: 847-674-7131 or 877-674-7131; e-mail: http://www.norfolkaccess.com; website: http://www.norfolkaccess.com).

2. Allentown Caging Equipment, Inc., Rt. 526, P.O. Box 698, Allentown, NJ 08501 (Telephone: 609-259-7951 or 800-762-2243; website: http://www.acecaging.com).

3. Alternative Design Manufacturing and Supply Company, 3055 Cheri Whitlock Drive, P.O. Box 6330 Siloam Springs, AR 72761 (Telephone: 479-524-4343 or 800-320-2459; e-mail: mail@altdesign.com; website: http://www.altdesign.com).

4. Alza Corporation, 1900 Charleston Road, P.O. Box 7210, Mountain View, CA 94039-7210 (Telephone: 650-564-5000; website: http://www.alza.com/).

5. Ancare Corporation, 2647 Grand Avenue, P.O. Box 814, Bellmore, NY 11710 (Telephone: 516-781-0755 or 800-645-6379; e-mail: information@ancare.com; website: http://www.ancare.com).

6. Bio-Serv, 1 8th St., Frenchtown, NJ 08825 (Telephone: 908-996-2155 or 800-996-9908; Fax: 908-996-4123; e-mail: sales@bio-serv.com; website: http://www.bio-serv.com).

7. Braintree Scientific, Inc., P.O. Box 850929, Braintree, MA 02185 (Telephone: 781-843-2202; e-mail: info@braintreesci.com; website: http://www.braintreesci.com).

8. Britz-Heidbrink, Inc., 1302 9th Street, Wheatland, WY 82201 (Telephone: 307-322-4040; e-mail: sales@BHenrich.com; website: http://www.BHenrich.com).

9. Burns Veterinary Supply, Inc., 1900 Diplomat Drive, Farmers Branch, TX 75234 (Telephone: 972-620-9941 or 800-922-8767; e-mail: http://burnsvet.com/scripts/contactus.asp; website: http://burnsvet.com).

10. Butler Animal Health Supply, LLC, 5600 Blazer Parkway, Dublin, OH 43017 (Telephone: 800-848-5983; website: https://www.accessbutler.com).

11. Colonial Medical Supply Company, Inc., 504 Wells Road, Franconia, NH 03580 (Telephone: 888-446-8427; e-mail: cms@colmedsupply.com; website: http://www.colmedsupply.com).

12. Fisher Scientific Inc., 711 Forbes Avenue, Pittsburgh, PA 15219-4785 (Telephone: 800-766-7000; website: www.fishersci.com).

13. Harvard Apparatus, Inc., 84 October Hill Road, Holliston, MA 01746 (Telephone: 508-893-8999 or 800-272-2775; e-mail: bioscience@harvardapparatus.com; website: www.harvardapparatus.com).

14. Instech Solomon, Inc., 5209 Militia Hill Road, Plymouth Meeting, PA 19462 (Telephone: 800-443-4227 or 610-941-0132; e-mail: support@.instechlabs.com; website: www.instechlabs.com.).

15. Lab Products, Inc., 742 Sussex Street, P.O. Box 639, Seaford, DE 19973 (Telephone: 302-628-4300 or 800-526-0469; website: http://www.labproductsinc.com).

16. Lenderking Caging Products, 8370 Jumpers Hole Road, Millersville, MD 21108 (Telephone: 410-544-8795; e-mail: sales@lenderking.com; website: http://www.lenderking.com).

17. LGL Animal Care Products, Inc., 1520 Cavitt Street, Bryan, TX 77801 (Telephone: 979-775-1776; e-mail: inform@lglacp.com; website: http://www.lglacp.com).

18. Lock Solutions, Inc., 12 Industrial Drive, P.O. Box 1099, Laurence Harbor, NJ 08879 (Telephone: 732-441-0982 or 800-947-0304; e-mail: locksolx3@aol.com).

19. Lomir Biomedical, Inc., 95 Huot, Notre-Dame Ile Perrot, Quebec, Canada J7V 7M4 (Telephone: 514-425-3604 or 877-425-3604; website: http://www.lomir.com).

20. Henry Schein, 135 Duryea Road, Melville, NY 11747 (Telephone: 631-843-5500 or 800-711-6032; e-mail: custserv@henryschein.com; website: www.henryschein.com).

21. Surburban Surgical Co., Inc., 275 12th Street, Wheeling, IL 60090 (Telephone: 847-537-9320 or 800-323-7366, ext. 3484; website: http://www.suburban-surgical.com).

22. SurgiVet/Anesco, N7 W22025 Johnson Road, Waukesha, WI 53186 (Telephone: 262-513-8500 or 888-745-6562; e-mail: sales@surgivet.com; website: http://www.surgivet.com).

23. Unifab Corporation, 5260 Lovers Lane, Portage, MI 49002 (Telephone: 269-382-2803 or 800-648-9569; website: www.unifab.com).

24. Viking Medical, P.O. Box 2142, Medford Lakes, NJ 08055 (Telephone: 800-920-1033; e-mail: info@vikingmedical.com; website: http://www.vikingmedical.com).

25. VWR International, 1310 Goshen Parkway, West Chester, PA 19380 (Telephone: 800-932-5000; website: http://www.vwrsp.com).

26. Webster Veterinary Supply, 86 Leominster Road, Sterling, MA 01564 (Telephone: 978-422-8211 or 800-225-7911; website: http://www.jawebster.com).

index

T - #0562 - 101024 - C0 - 234/156/10 - PB - 9780849328930 - Gloss Lamination